CANCER CAREGIVER ROLES:
What You Need to Know

Medical and Scheduling Support
Insurance Management
Home Care Management

Pay It Forward
When you are through with this book, please PASS IT ON
to someone you know who has been diagnosed with cancer.

ISBN: 978-1-4525-5346-7 (sc)
ISBN: 978-1-4525-5345-0 (e)

Balboa Press books may be ordered through booksellers or by contacting:

Balboa Press
A Division of Hay House
1663 Liberty Drive
Bloomington, IN 47403
www.balboapress.com
1-(877) 407-4847

Because of the dynamic nature of the Internet, any web addresses or links contained in this book may have changed since publication and may no longer be valid. The views expressed in this work are solely those of the author and do not necessarily reflect the views of the publisher, and the publisher hereby disclaims any responsibility for them.

The author of this book does not dispense medical advice or prescribe the use of any technique as a form of treatment for physical, emotional, or medical problems without the advice of a physician, either directly or indirectly. The intent of the author is only to offer information of a general nature to help you in your quest for emotional and spiritual well-being. In the event you use any of the information in this book for yourself, which is your constitutional right, the author and the publisher assume no responsibility for your actions.

Printed in the United States of America

Balboa Press rev. date: 12/31/2012

Representations

This book was compiled and published under the auspices of Family Caregiving, LLC: Improving Patient Care by Improving Family Caregiving.

The views and statements made in this book are solely those of the author. The author acknowledges that he is not an oncologist, an attorney, nor an accountant. The author is not providing medical, legal, or accounting opinions or conclusions. This is information he personally gathered, developed and utilized during his late wife's nine year battle with cancer.

The sole purpose of this book is to assist other family caregivers who may find themselves in a similar situation with a loved one who is fighting cancer or an end of life situation.

Nothing herein is to be construed as a solicitation; that is not the intent of the author.

Profits from the sale of this book will be donated to Hospice and to Cancer research.

It is strongly recommended that the reader contact an attorney, or an accountant, or a member of the patient's Oncology Team with reference to any questions concerning information provided in this book

BALBOA
PRESS
A DIVISION OF HAY HOUSE

DEDICATION

**This book is dedicated to cancer patient Family Caregivers ---
that exhausting, noble, deepest expression of human love.**

It was also written to honor my loved one, Susan Marie, deceased after a nine year battle with breast cancer that spread into her spine, and finally into her brain. Susan was a great teacher, from whom I have learned everything that is important in my life. She also taught me that Family Caregiving is truly a sacred calling. This work is my way to give her struggles, her gifts, and her memory to the readers of this book. May she teach and inspire *them* to become more loving and proficient in their new life journey together.

CANCER CAREGIVER ROLES

PREFACE

"You have cancer........." These words hit us like a thunderbolt, out of the blue. We struggled to comprehend what was said. Our minds imploded in disbelief; our thoughts became incomprehensible....numb disconnects. And a gnawing primal fear began to well up in our hearts. These are arguably the three most dreaded words in life.

"You have cancer........." means that TWO LIVES are going to change ---one becoming now the life of a cancer patient, and the other the life of the caregiving partner. You are both now about to embark on a new, evolving, and life-changing journey, that deeply engages both of you in the coming months and years. You have just entered into a new phase in your partnership relationship: between husband and wife, between offspring and parent, between caregiver and patient.

As time goes by, more effort will needed to keep up with all the support processes; the caregiver's involvement gets deeper and deeper, until it threatens to consume the entire energy and soul of the caregiver.

The caregiver must re-prioritize *what can be done* to keep everything as close to "normal" as possible. But family and household matters must be balanced by work necessities and ever increasing physiological and emotional caregiving requirements. A "new normal" will have to evolve and be established and accepted by both partners.

Soon, three *specific new support roles* will emerge for the caregiving partner:

1) **Medical Support**—including scheduling, medication support, monitoring side effects, managing pain, maintaining medical records, and advance medical directives;

2) **Insurance and Financial Management**—selecting the right insurance plans to cover the new and expensive cancer drugs, or finding resources if there is no insurance, and saving you both from financial devastation;

3) **Household Management**—including nutrition management, safety, controls for infection, as well as providing physical/emotional/spiritual support.

Cancer is a disease that affects *both* of you—changing your lives, changing your focus, changing your priorities. Cancer gives new purpose to each partner, a new mission. Under these new conditions, *each person's life now gives new meaning and new purpose to the other partner, and to the bond between them.*

Cancer always involves TWO.

LEARN AS MUCH AS YOU CAN, as QUICKLY as you can.

Unless you are a Physician or Registered Nurse, as a layman you will need to learn new terminology and a new way of talking about your loved one's experiences with her disease. You will have to learn to wade through a new language. The cancer caregiver must learn a new vocabulary to be able to understand what is going on with their loved one, and to work intelligently with the Medical Teams.

Cancer has opened up a new world, into which the caregiver needs to find comfort, intelligence and mobility. This is especially true in the new role of Monitor of Side Effects. The caregiver needs to 'expatriate" from his comfort zone or what has been his usual business life and become embedded in understanding a strange new world of medical terminology and relationships. Being a great caregiver demands this, just like a business assignment to a foreign country requires one to be open and *absorb the new culture* of that foreign country.

This document is my effort to share my caregiving experiences within my own cancer partner, in the hope that they will help the readers anticipate and cope with the new realities in their lives.

Becoming a good caregiver is a daunting task, requiring your full capabilities effort, and creativity. Both of you will learn from each other: new levels of giving, new levels of heart, new levels of purpose, new ways of thinking, new levels of togetherness, new levels of Being: ***physically, intellectually, emotionally, and spiritually.***

......Bon Voyage

1) Definitions:

Cancer: There are more than 200 types of cancer distinguished into general categories of _liquid_ cancers [leukemia (blood), lymphoma (lymph system), myeloma (plasma/bone)] and _solid cancers_ which appear as a cell mass, clump, or tumor [including breast cancer, skin cancer, lung cancer, colon cancer, prostate cancer, liver cancer, pancreatic cancer, brain cancer, bone cancer… etc].   Cancer symptoms vary widely based on the type and level of development of the cancer in the body.

The word "cancer" comes from the Greek word _karkinos_ or "crab." Cancer is characterized by the uncontrolled growth of a group of mutated normal cells ("tumors") that reach out crab-like infecting surrounding healthy cells.

Not all tumors are cancerous. A _benign_ tumor (or kind tumor) is not cancerous; benign tumors tend to grow more slowly and their cells tend to stay together.   A _malignant_ tumor (or evil tumor) is made up of abnormal cells that divide rapidly or uncontrollably and invade nearby healthy cells or migrate to another organ or another part of the body.

Cancer is fundamentally a genetic disease. _Cancer begins by a single cell undergoing genetic mutation and dividing to form two mutated cells, who divide…and divide….etc., finally becoming malignant cancer cells expressing mutations that signal uncontrolled cell growth and adaptation, and mutations that inhibit signals to suppress cell growth or signal death to the cell._ To use an automobile analogy: the gear shift breaks off stuck in "Drive" sending a constant signal to the transmission to engage forward motion; similarly brake fluid has drained out from a leak in the brake line, and even if you step on the brake pedal you are unable to signal the brakes to suppress the forward movement. _Cancer is stuck in "Drive" and the brakes don't work._

But this happens in stages—mutations are very rare occurrences.   Fully malignant Cancer usually grows slowly taking years or decades to emerge; someone can smoke all their life but the malignant tumor doesn't appear until old age.   It depends on how quickly the gene mutations occur and the type of cancer involved. Advanced cancer usually results from prolonged _metastases_ (spread) where the cancer just takes over entire parts of the body, beginning to limit the life expectancy of the cancer patient.

Cancer tumors become mutated versions of healthy cells, and consequent mutations allow the tumor to travel through the blood or the lymph systems (_metastasize_) spreading to colonize and infect other tissues or organs. Another characteristic allows the cancerous cells to draw blood vessels to themselves to provide the cancer tumor with nutrition (_angiogenesis_). Still another adaptation excretes any toxic or waste substances from within the cell, an adaptation rendering medications like chemotherapy to ultimately become ineffective. Cancer cells are just truncated but perverted versions of our healthy selves using the same functional cellular mechanisms to survive.

[Sources: www.ted.com click talks, search cancer.   Siddhartha Mukherjee, The Emperor of all Maladies,-- Pulitzer Prize winning history of cancer told through biographies of the major physicians and researchers of the last 4000 years.]

Oncology: (from the Ancient Greek *onkos*, meaning *bulk, mass, burden,* or *tumor*), is a branch of medicine that deals with malignant tumors or cancer. A medical professional who practices oncology is an *oncologist*.

To confirm the cancer diagnosis, a *biopsy* is performed, where a tissue sample is analyzed under a microscope to determine if it exhibits cancerous growth.

Cancer Stages: When cancer is originally diagnosed or later when tests are run to determine levels of development or remission, the stage of development is generally described by one of the following agreed upon characteristics. Generally, the earlier the cancer stage, the better the treatment prognosis:

Stage 1 —small cancer tumor found only in the organ where it started.

Stage 2 —larger cancer tumor that may or may not have spread to the lymph nodes. Cancer cells can spread through the body through the vascular (blood) system, or the lymphatic system. If surgery is performed, some "sentinel" lymph nodes can be analyzed to see if any cancer cells have moved into the lymph system.

Stage 3 —larger cancer tumor that is also in the lymph nodes.

Stage 4 —metastasized cancer found in a different organ or tissue from where it started; usually named by the organ or tumor of origin (e.g., breast cancer spread to the pelvis is still called metastatic breast cancer.....etc)

Tumors in this Stage 4 are more aggressive, requiring stronger treatment regimens.

Diagnostics

Early detection of cancer can lead to early treatment, and this greatly improves a person's chances of surviving the disease.

Most tumors are discovered when a medical professional or the Patient notices signs or symptoms and reports them to a medical provider: a technician may discover an abnormality in a mammogram, or the Patient may feel an odd lump or notice blood in the stool. Routine physical exams and/or screenings are also a good source of early detection.

Biopsy: Once the abnormality is suspected, the first step in making the medical determination whether a tumor is *benign* or *malignant* involves the removal of a small number of cells or tissue for study under a microscope: ***biopsy***. A biopsy can determine if the cells are cancerous, as well as determine exactly what type of cancer is present.

X-rays: X-rays are a form of electromagnetic radiaiton that can penetrate clothing, body tissue, and internal organs. An X-ray machine sends this radiation through the body. Some of the radiation emerges on the other side of the body, where it exposes film or is absorbed by a digital detector to create an image. And some of it is absorbed in body tissues as it goes through. Radiation is painless; but larger doses, as received in Radiation Oncology can create skin irritation or abrasions, and longer term side effects. Radiation directed at the tumor kills cancer cells; but it also affects any fast-growth healthy cells in the region. For example, radiation of the head is directed at destroying cancer cells, but it also can kill the follicles of the hair, making hair loss permanent.

CT Scans, or CAT Scans: Computed Tomography [CT] is a new form of imaging using X-rays. Whereas, X-rays create a two-dimensional image, a CT Scan produces cross-sectional or three-dimensional view of a part of thee body by passing several X-ray beams through the body from different angles, and then using a computer to restructure the information into the shape of a 3-D picture. CT scans can be done with or without an injection of an intravenous contrast dye, which helps the physician or technician to see facets of the tumor. Following the CT scan, a patient is encouraged to drink fluids to promote the excretion of the dye. Nearly *half* of all medical X-ray exposures today come from CT equipment, and radiation doses from CT are higher than other X-ray studies.
Tell your Oncologist or CT Technician if you have an allergy to iodine or shellfish.

[Source: National Council on Radiation Protection and Measurements]

Magnetic Resonance Imaging [MRI]:   MRI is somewhat like an x-ray but it is more detailed. An MRI provides multiplane, cross-sectional images of whatever part of the body is being targeted. MRI technology is based on the magnetism in certain cells in the human body, and their interaction with radio waves.

There is no radiation exposure. The only discomfort may be from lying on a narrow hard surface in a confined "tube." A patient may experience tingling in metal teeth fillings as well as a constant heavy rumble and ticking sound during the procedure. The procedure may take anywhere from 15 minutes to up to 60 minutes. An anti-anxiety medication may be needed for those with mild claustrophobia.

Positron Emission Tomography [PET]:   PET scanning provides information about the body's chemistry not available through other procedures. Unlike CT (computerized tomography) or MRI (magnetic resonance imaging) techniques that look at anatomy or body form, PET studies *metabolic activity* or body *function*. PET has been used primarily in cardiology, neurology, and oncology.

In PET the patient receives a short half-lived radioactive substance. The amount of radiation exposure the patient receives is about the same as two chest X-rays.

PET enables the physician to see the location of metabolic processes. The scanners electronics point out locations where metabolic functions are occurring. For example, glucose (or sugar, which the body uses to produce energy) combined with a radioisotope will show where glucose is being metabolized in the brain, the heart muscle, or a growing tumor. PET enables the doctor or technician to locate tumor activity, and this technology is frequently used with x-rays or CT scans for purposes of comparison.

Endoscopy: Endoscopy is a broad term used to described examining the inside of the patient's body using a *lighted, flexible* tube called an endoscope through which the lining of the esophagus, stomach, and duodenum can be viewed using a TV monitor. In general, an endoscope is introduced into the body through a natural opening like the mouth or anus. Although endoscopy can include examination of other organs, the most common endoscopic procedures evaluate the esophagus, duodenum, stomach, and upper portions of the intestine. A variation, called *colonoscopy*, inserts the endoscope through the rectum and provides visualization of the large intestine.

Another variation is *bronchoscopy* where the fiberoptic tube is inserted down the throat for direct inspection of the larynx, trachea and lungs. Tissue samples can be obtained and secretions collected through the tube for study or biopsy. Numbing medicine or a partial anesthesia is given to the patient to help them relax during the procedure.

Capsule endoscopy is a very new technology that uses a swallowed video capsule to take photographs of the inside of the esophagus, stomach, and small intestine.   As the capsule travels through the esophagus, stomach, and small intestine, it takes photographs rapidly. The photographs are transmitted by the radio transmitter to a small receiver that is worn on the waist of the patient who is undergoing the capsule endoscopy. At the end of the procedure, approximately 24 hours later, the photographs are downloaded from the receiver into a computer, and the images are reviewed by a physician. The capsule is passed by the patient into the toilet and flushed away.

Untrasonography: An utrasound procedure is a diagnostic test in which high-frequency sound waves are bounced off tissues or a tumor and the **echoes are converted into a picture** (sonogram). Most popular in its use to see a fetus in its developmental stages. Ultrasound technology provides no exposure to radiation, is noninvasive, and painless. A *gel* is applied topically to the skin above the area being examined which will enhance sound transmission.

Fine Needle Aspiration [FNA]: FNA is a method of inserting a thin needle directly into the mass or tumor, and cells are removed for examination under a microscopy by a pathologist, the medical specialty that deals with making diagnoses of diseases and conditions through the examination of cell samples from the body.

Usually conducted in the Examination Room on felt breast masses, FNA can be performed on any felt tumor in the body. For most individuals there is minimal discomfort and Preliminary Results may be immediately available.

Diagnostic Imaging and diagnostic testing have given the medical practitioner new and powerful tools that enable the professional to actually _see_ what is going on inside the body. This information then greatly assists the selection of the appropriate treatment for the specific tumor, and patient-specific treatments can be developed.

With the upcoming era of genetics and genetic testing, medical practitioners will be enabled to extend their knowledge of the specific patient, including the identification of future disease risks; the *prediction of drug responses*; and the detection of risks of disease to future children

Treatments

Medical Oncology:

Surgery:

Medical Oncology treats cancer from the perspective of cancer drugs *(chemotherapy)* which are intended to retard the growth of the tumor, or to kill cancer cells without also destroying too many adjacent healthy cells.

Medical oncology also engages the surgical removal of the cancerous tumor, if it is determined that this treatment will be effective. The first line of attack against a specific malignant tumor is to determine if it can be surgically removed [removed or excised = "...ectomy; " to remove a lump = "lumpectomy,"to remove a breast = "mastectomy"].

Chemotherapy:

While surgery is specific to the tumor and its surroundings, chemotherapy is *systemic*, affecting the cells of the entire body, consequently impacting *healthy cells* that are also fast-growing or which divide rapidly. Normal cells that will be affected include *hair follicles*, consequently cancer patients taking chemotherapy frequently lose their hair, *gastrointestinal tract cells* leading to diarrhea, nausea, or constipation, cells of the *bone marrow*, leading to low blood counts and extreme fatigue, and some *reproductive organ* cells, leading to low sperm counts and infertility. Although hair loss will usually occur about two weeks after the initial chemo treatment, hair loss is reversible and will normally grow back within a few months after the last treatment. Most patients plan ahead and obtain a wig or hats, scarves or turbans. The American Cancer Society has a free wig boutique that may be helpful to the patient: 1.800.227.2345, open 24 hours a day.

A fairly recent approach to fighting cancer cells by using the body's natural immune system is called "Biotherapy" or sometimes "Immunotherapy." One of the agents commonly used in this therapy is Herceptin (trastuzumab) which can be used in combination with other chemo drugs, or as a stand-alone medication.
These drugs are biological hormone receptor inhibitors which interrupt the supply of nutrients to the cancer cells.

As the Caregiver Partner of a Cancer Patient, it is extremely important to remember that chemotherapy may affect the marrow of your loved one's bones leading to low blood counts especially of the white blood cells. This makes your loved one much more susceptible to infections.
Personal hygiene actions become extremely important—especially frequent *WASHING OF HANDS.*   [See discussion in Section 25: Controls for Infection.]

Radiation Oncology:

Radiation Oncology involves the use of powerful x-ray beams to destroy cancer cells. Radiation therapy can target and kill cells, or change their ability to divide and multiply, with lower risk of permanently injuring adjacent normal cells. The high energy beams are streams of particles generated by a special machine called a linear accelerator.

Radiation therapy is usually divided into several daily treatments and dosage is carefully planned to limit the exposure of healthy tissue.

X-ray beams can be broadly focused such as in whole-head radiation, or radiation beams can be pinpointed directly onto the tumor itself.

An advanced form of pinpointed radiation has recently become available called *Stereotactic Radiosurgery*. In this latter form of radiation, multiple beams of radiation are directed through the body at many different angles *converging* with pinpoint accuracy to blast the targeted tumor with cumulative energy. This procedure minimizes side effects and collateral damage of surrounding healthy tissue and skin. Stereotactic Radiosurgery can accomplish in fewer procedures, what was previously expected from longer conventional radiation treatment protocols.

At other times, tiny radioactive pellets are inserted inside the tumor, and work to destroy the tumor from the inside out; this is called "brachytherapy." Sometimes these pellets are inserted into the area around an incision where a cancer tumor has been removed by surgery, to kill any tumor cells that may remain.

Radiation therapy may also be used to shrink a tumor before surgery, or to relieve symptoms of cancer like pressure, bleeding, or pain.

The planning process is quite complex, involving selecting the correct beam sizes, angles, energies, and shielding for the body. Treatments will then require the Patient to assume a fixed position, so devices such as molds, masks and blocks may be used to maintain the position. Although the Patient will be alone in the treatment room, he/she will be monitored continuously and he/she can converse with the therapists via intercom. The machine will perform all the motion necessary to aim the beam from the predetermined angles.

There is no pain other than discomfort from the hardness of the table and the immobility required. After treatments, the patient can go back to daily routines.

The patient will be monitored for skin irritations from the radiation; and we learned that whole-head radiation can permanently damage or kill hair follicles, and hair will not return in the area radiated.

Markers

Tumor markers are substances that can be detected in higher-than-normal amounts in the blood, urine, or body tissues of some patients with certain types of cancer. A tumor marker may be made by a tumor itself or by the body in response to the tumor.

Although tumor markers are typically imperfect as screening tests to detect occult (hidden) cancers, once a particular tumor has been found *the marker may be used as an indicator for monitoring the success or failure of treatment.* The tumor marker level may also reflect the extent or the stage of the disease, indicate how quickly the cancer is likely to progress and so help determine the prognosis.

CA 27-29:   A marker that is found in the blood of most breast cancer patients. CA 27-29 levels may be used in conjunction with other procedures (such as mammograms and measurements of other tumor marker levels) to check for recurrence in women previously treated for stage II and stage III breast cancer. CA 27-29 levels can also be elevated by cancers of the colon, stomach, kidney, lung, ovary, pancreas, uterus, and liver.

CA 125 is a protein that is a so-called biomarker, which is a substance that is found in greater concentration in tumor cells than in other cells of the body. In particular, CA 125 is present in greater concentration in *ovarian cancer* cells than in other cells.

CEA [Carcinoembryonic Antigen] is a protein found in many types of cells but associated with tumors in the body and fetus growth. CEA is tested in blood. The main use of CEA is as a tumor marker, especially with intestinal cancer. The most common cancers that elevate CEA are in the colon and rectum. Others: pancreas, stomach, lung, breast and certain types of thyroid cancer. CEA levels over 20 ng/ml are associated with cancer which has already metastasized (spread). A rising CEA level indicates progression or recurrence of the cancer. CEA is useful in monitoring the treatment of CEA-rich tumors; if the CEA is high before treatment, it should fall to normal [< 5.0 ng/ml] after successful therapy.

  It would be wise for the Caregiver to become familiar with the particular marker associated with the type of cancer diagnosed for the Patient. You can then participate in following or "tracking" the effects of treatment, or conversely the growth of cancer reflected in the blood stream. These are not exact measures, but rather an indicator of the directions taken by the disease. You can trace the general progression or containment of your loved one's cancer by following these markers or indicators.

[See column number 6 of Lab Results, **Exhibit 2b**.]

Clinical Trials: Clinical trials are research studies in which people help oncologists or researchers
improve the care of cancer patients. These studies try to answer scientific questions or try to find better ways to prevent, diagnose and treat the disease. Clinical trials try to determine whether a specific drug or treatment regimen is safe and effective for the treatment of a specific condition. Clinical Trials go through three phases:

Phase I: Researchers try to evaluate the *safety* of a new medicine or treatment, the *best dose* or schedule to be used in the treatment, and what types of *side effects* occur.

Phase II: The medicine or treatment is tested on a larger group with the disease in question, and researchers try to ascertain *how well* the medicine or treatment works with respect to a particular medical condition.

Phase III: Tested on an even larger group, now the medicine or treatment is studied to find out how well it works compared to standard treatments or placebo. During this phase, patients are given the study medicine or treatment, the standard treatment , and a placebo on a randomized basis. Most medicines that reach Phase 3 trials are considered for FDA approval.

Phase IV: Tests are now conducted to find new uses for the medicine, or new ways of administering it, or
any additional safety information. For example: it may be studied on a specific population cohort or demographic like how well it works on adults over 65, or a specific racial group.

Risks:
- The new treatment may not work as well as standard treatments.
- Your loved one may experience serious or even life-threatening side effects.
- The trial may take up more time than standard treatments.

Most insurance carriers will not pay for your loved one to participate in a Clinical Trial; however, normally all the costs of treatment are covered by the organization sponsoring the Trial.

If you have an interest in pursuing this for your loved one, ***begin by consulting your Medical Oncologist..***

Also you may wish to consult <www.ClinicalTrials.gov> which is a web site developed by the National Library of Medicine of the U.S. National Institutes of Health to provide information about clinical research to the public.

Intravenous Port: As cancer regresses or progresses, your loved one has experienced continuous injections of chemotherapy, ancillary drugs, fluids, and blood draws—each involving a "needle prick" to locate and insert the syringe into a vein.

After a time, the veins of the arm and hand become so bruised and sore, as well as abuse from the toxic drugs that have been infused into them, that your loved one should consider asking for a Port.

In medicine, a Port (or portacath) is a small medical appliance that is surgically inserted into the upper chest or arm and appears as a bump under the skin. The device requires no special maintenance and is completely inserted under the skin, so bathing or swimming are not a problem.

The Port consists of a small reservoir compartment with a silicone bubble for needle insertion (the septum), with an attached plastic tube (catheter) that is inserted into a vein. This allows infused medications to be spread quickly and efficiently throughout the body. The Port may also be used to draw blood from the vein. The Port provides vein access with minimal discomfort—much less than the typical "needle stick."

ASK YOUR ONCOLOGIST or Infusion RN about information that is available to help you make the decision whether or not to proceed with this option. Check with others in the Infusion area and get their opinion about the usefulness and convenience of having a Port.

Our experience was **extremely positive** once the port was inserted. It was virtually painless, it gave us a much easier way to obtain blood draws, or infuse drugs or chemotherapy. It was easy to keep clean, and did not bother her showering. It was not visible under clothing. My wife's arms and veins cleared up and regained healthy vascular function. We several times questioned why we had not done this earlier in her cancer journey.

---

2) **Office Appointments:**

 It is not fun to go see a doctor; but when your loved one is afflicted with a progressive and degenerative disease, it becomes a necessity to preserve continuity of treatment and ultimately, to prolong life itself.

It is useful to combine your insurance cards with your State Driver's License and to keep these together in a wallet or purse. An ID Lanyard that hangs around your neck allows you to openly wear the identifying documents, much like the ID document you may find pinned to your Physician's shirt, or hanging from around his/her neck. Hospitals use these highly visible ID Lanyards to easily identify the person wearing them and be able to validate their ability to come and go.

In filling out the usual *Patient Admission Form* for any new Physician, you will always be asked for a LIST OF THE MEDICATIONS your Partner is taking on a daily routine basis, or as needed on a specific schedule or on an occasional basis.. It is a huge time saver to produce an updated a Patient List of Medications and this helps any new Physician to make informed decisions in any new circumstance. This is one of the most *useful* documents that can be produced; it will be used continuously.

I learned to carry about 6 – 10 copies of the *Patient Medications Lists* in my loved one's Medical Folder and they were constantly updated every time there was a change in medication or dosing.

[To see an *actual Patient Medications List*, See **Exhibit 1a and Exhibit 1b**]

 Normal procedure of an Office Appointment begins with Check-In, and then WEIGHT, BLOOD PRESSURE, and OXYGENATION measurements. As a Caregiving Partner, it is useful to keep a log of WEIGHT, as a marker for how well the PATIENT's nutritional needs are being met, and BLOOD PRESSURE as an indicator of overall STRESS effects and overall well-being. These measurements are usually entered into the patient's Medical Records but are not given to the Patient or Caregiver unless they have been requested.

 Also, it is a good practice to request a Patient Copy of the results of any of the DIAGNOSTIC IMAGING PROCEDURES, and BLOOD DRAWS. These will be helpful to understand how the Patient is progressing, and useful if your Patient has to go to see another Specialist or Oncologist.

[See **Exhibit 2a** and **Exhibit 2b**]

---

3) Calendar Management :

Breaking up the normal cancer routines is always hard on both the Caregiving Partner and the Cancer Patient; transportation must be arranged, usually the Patient must dress to go out, which also might include bathing or clean up.

It is very difficult—like herding cats—to obtain multiple appointments from different Physician Offices if you have to meet with more than one physician or more than one location, but the effort is worth attempting for the Patient's sake if the outcome is multiple visits in the same day. It may also help the Patient's emotional and physical recovery to complete the hassle and travel of all these visits.

But the lesson of this section is OBTAIN A CALENDAR , DAYTIMER, or Calendar your schedule on your Laptop, cell or I-Phone. It is very difficult to reschedule an overlooked or forgotten appointment, sometimes taking months to find the next opening in the Physician's schedule.

Another use of this Office Visit record is for VERIFICATION when you receive the Explanation of Benefits [EOB] from your insurance company. The first column on the insurance company EOB is the "DATE of SERVICE" provided to your Patient Partner. I noted a discrepancy on the insurance company EOB indicating that Service was recorded to have been provided at one downtown hospital location at the same time that chemotherapy treatment was being provided at a Cancer Clinic in another town. Upon investigation, the Service Provided was coded to show a visit to the birthing unit of the hospital. It turned out to be a coding and posting error from the hospital, but it was worth several thousand dollars to our family as the insured party.

Computers in Accounting Departments can make mistakes.
It is important to have a permanent calendar record for verification when you look over your medical insurance records.

A final matter related to Calendar Management, is that you may need a record of the number of times and location where treatments were received FOR INCOME TAX PURPOSES. Mileage to and from a medical treatment is a deductible medical expense, and you may need your calendar as a record of your medical treatments, as information you can use to assist you to find evidentiary receipts for this deduction.

4) Timing / Dosage of Medication--Implementing the treatment plan at Home:

The Caregiver is the arm's length extension of your Oncologist and Oncology Team—at your loved one's home,--24/7.

 If you and your Patient Partner are on regimens of treatments, you will notice things like the need to ingest multiple pills at different times during the day. At one point, my Cancer Partner was consuming 16 different capsules, at different times during the day: Tykerb in the morning before breakfast, supplemental vitamins with breakfast, anti-inflamatory steroids at four intervals during the day, and antidpressants and sleep aids in the evening, with an occasional nausea drug, or drug for diarrhea,and/or a pain suppressant.

 My Partner found it very useful to use *3 Weekly Pill Boxes* that can be obtained at any commercial Pharmacy, or even grocery store. These separate pill boxes by day of the week: S M T W Th F S. We used one for early morning capsules, another for pills to be taken during the day, and the other to hold pills to be taken in the evening before bedtime. It was ESSENTIAL for keeping the pills sorted, and related to the time they were to be ingested.

 If you do not use pill boxes to sort your medications, IT IS ESSENTIAL **to record and check-off what was taken, and when it was taken.** THIS IS EXTREMELY IMPORTANT, if the Caregiver has to leave the home and go to work, being absent when these medications must be ingested. It is vital for the Patient not to "forget" what has been taken, and maybe even overdose by taking more than prescribed of these extremely strong medications. This could easily become a *life threatening situation*, if not handled accurately and seriously.

 Keep the weekly pill boxes to sort out meds for each day, but it is also important to develop a Schedule of Medications to see what has been ingested and what is yet to come.

My Partner used a White Board to record what and when meds were ingested. When meds changed, it was easy to erase the old and write in the new. It did not serve well as a permanent record.   A check-off system, laid out by DAY, AND TIME OF DAY, gives you the permanent record needed.

[See Meds Log, **Exhibit 3**]

```
┌─────────────────────────────────────────────────────┐
│                                                       │
│         CAREGIVER MEDICAL SUPPORT ROLES               │
│                                                       │
└─────────────────────────────────────────────────────┘
```

5)   Learning About the Medications:

The Caregiving Partner NEEDS TO BE INFORMED about the medications he is administering to his cancer Partner for *two critically important reasons*:

      1)   the Caregiving Partner needs to be the **Monitor of SIDE EFFECTS** for the Cancer Patient.

> Assume the Cancer Patient is suffering from diarrhea, or nausea, and terrible headaches after a round to chemotherapy treatment.   The Cancer Patient is in no condition to assess whether or not the situation is critical and a run to the Emergency Room or call to your Oncologist is warranted.

> But to make this decision, the Caregiver needs to be INFORMED of the potential side effects and their severity that are listed in the pharmacological description of the medication.   Ask questions, get help; but ultimately you are the only one who is home alone face-to-face with your loved one.

Where does the Caregiving Partner get this information?

The informational sources I found most helpful were:

      a) *the Internet*—{see the sources listed in order of informational importance and ease of understanding as **Exhibit 4**—especially useful were the sources listed as Five Star. I would encourage Caregivers to become familiar with the formats and information of: WebMD, MedicineNet, and the American Cancer Society <cancer.org>.

      b) the **pharmacological description** of any medication **provided by the Pharmacy** along with your prescription; these are very informative, including the side effects.

If the Caregiver or Patient have questions, or cannot reach the Oncologist, a call to the Pharmacist where the prescription was filled may be very helpful .   Remember, you are not alone. Your Oncologist, or Nurse Practitioner, or Pharmacist are there to be of help. But, do not hesitate to seek help---your loved one depends on it.

2) The Caregiver needs to be INFORMED to be able to provide helpful information or ask intelligent questions in meetings with the Oncologist or Oncology Team.   The Caregiver needs to become the semi-pro Home Nursing player to be useful to the Oncologist, the Team and to his loved one.

 Many times your Patient will not be in an alert physical or mental condition to follow and understand the Office conversations, and formulate questions.   Your loved one relies on YOU to figure what needs to be asked. The Caregiver may surely want to make notes during the meetings for reference at home later in the week.

It is sometimes hard to remember and transfer the technical directions given in the Oncologist's office back home, where the passage of days obscures your clarity of understanding that you seemed to experience in the office. Taking notes is essential.

The Caregiver is in a unique position to help the Oncology Team to fully understand the full holistic needs of their Patient.   Remember, your Oncologist may see your loved one or two times a month (with additional time for thinking, recording notes and research); but you *live with* your Patient --24/7.

The Caregiver plays a crucial role here. **You** must implement the day-to-day parts of the oncology treatment plan. Long time direct contact and full time, full range assistance of your loved one can greatly support and inform the Medical Team and improve your loved one's quality of care.

DO NOT BE AFRAID TO SPEAK UP.

A recent study, concluded May 20, 2010, by the Feinberg School of Medicine of Northwestern University fully acknowledges the critical informational role the Caregiver plays in keeping the Oncology Team informed.

 The findings of the study show that patients with brain tumors very often tend to be overly optimistic in reporting their condition to the Oncology Team. Whether they actually feel that way, or are just fed up with treatments and want to avoid continued or new regimens of treatment is not conclusive, But the Team is fully dependent upon the Caregiver to clearly describe and report the real extent of the Patient's cancer condition and symptoms.

> [See Study : Feinberg School of Medicine, Northwestern Univ.
> *Quality of Life Concordance between Patients....and their*
> *Caregivers,* funded by Am. Brain Tumor Association]

----

6) Managing Pain:

Cancer patients experience pain. Pain may be tumor related, or experienced from immobility, or joint pain, or muscle atrophy. Relief prevents suffering, and may help the Patient heal faster. Pain can affect every aspect off your loved one's Quality of Life: activity, appetite, sleep, energy, mood, relationships. Pain can be **acute** (sudden, localized) or become **chronic**.   For chronic pain, it may be best to take pain medications on a schedule that anticipates and prevents the pain from coming on.

How to report Pain:

1)   <u>How it feels</u>: "achy, ""throbbing,"" burning, ""stabbing," "pressure............"

2)   <u>How much pain do you have?</u>

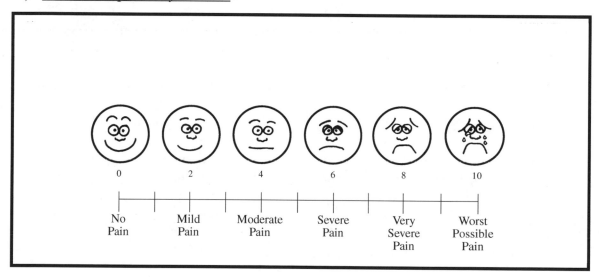

0	2	4	6	8	10
No Pain	Mild Pain	Moderate Pain	Severe Pain	Very Severe Pain	Worst Possible Pain

If you are unable to describe the level of pain you are experiencing by a number like "I have a very painful headache—about a 7 or an 8---" try using words like "mild" "moderate" or "severe."   At least try to describe for your Caregiver or the Oncologist **WHERE** you feel pain, and tell **WHEN** it started, and **WHAT** makes you feel worse, or better.

<u>**Do not be afraid to report pain to the Oncology Team**</u>. <u>They will take your loved one</u> <u>seriously and try to come up with solutions that will ease your loved one's pain and make her feel</u> <u>better.</u>

Pain can usually be controlled by the use of pain medications. Normally these depend upon the source, and degree of pain expressed.

Severe Pain is best treated with narcotics like morphine or Fentanyl, or Oxycodone. These are only available *by prescription* from your Pharmacy, and can develop side effects like severe constipation. The patient should drink plenty of fluids and eat foods high in fiber, such as fruits or brans. Narcotic drugs can be habit forming, and this needs to be monitored.

Mild to Moderate Pain is usually treated with over-the-counter medications like Tylenol or Aleve, or non-steroidal anti-inflammatory (NSAIDs) like aspirin or Advil (ibuprofen). Sometimes a *sedative* like Ativan can help relieve pain while it focuses on relief of anxiety for your loved one.

Learn as much as you can about HOW your loved one expresses pain nonverbally. Is she restless? groaning,? breathing heavily? face wrinkled up? jaw tight? fists clenched?

Over the last two years of my loved one's life, I carefully observed her habits and idiosyncrasies, and learned to distinguish when she was *signaling anxiety* (which is treated by sedatives such as *Ativan*) or *signaling pain* (which is treated by narcotics, or Aleve, or Ibuprophens).

She would raise a hand to her jaw or cheek for anxiety, and tighten fists or put her hands over her chest (sternum), because the cancer in her spine could not be pinpointed by her any more than just pain somewhere behind her chest.

This information became very useful in her end-of-life care at Pathways Hospice, where she ultimately became *unable to verbally communicate* with her caregivers.

---

7) <u>MONITORING SIDE EFFECTS: one of Caregiver's most important medical roles.</u>

By law, pharmacological descriptions of all drugs must *list* Side Effects. The problem for the layman is that *ALL SIDE EFFECTS* that were experienced in the testing and clinical trials of the drug must be listed, and it becomes difficult for the Caregiver to know **which to take most seriousl**y and which may be incidental or less critical to the Patient's wellbeing.   Many times, the pharmacological report will differentiate "regular" or "usual" Side Effects, and then the Report will list CAUTIONS about two or three "severe" or even "life threatening" Side Effects. Pay close attention to the latter. <u>These are situations where *what you don't know* can severely injure your Partner.</u>

For example, *diarrhea* is one of the primary side effects of the chemo drug Lapatinib.   If diarrhea becomes severe, lasts more than 48 or 72 hours after medication, or if the Patient *shows signs of severe dehydration such as severe dizziness or decreased amount of urine,* the Oncologist or Pharmacist should be called immediately.

<u>Understand that your loved one is GOING THROUGH THE EXPERIENCE of side effects, and just may not be capable of assessing their negative consequences, or implications for treatment modification.</u>   Your loved one just feels miserable and just wants relief.

The Caregiver must take on the responsibility to know **what to expect** from a treatment, and have enough INFORMATION to make assessments, after learning about cautions and severity of side effects, to be able to make the choices *WHEN TO MAKE THE CALL*, or *WHEN TO GET THEIR LOVED ONE INTO THE CAR* for a run to the Clinic, Cancer Center, or the Hospital Emergency Room,

---

A possibly confusing issue that may give trouble to the family home caregiver, who is swimming in unfamiliar waters, is in the labeling of the chemo drugs.

<u>Medicine gives two names to each drug:</u>

       1) the first label is the name of the drug class or the drug's <u>GENERIC NAME</u>—in the case of the previous paragraph, the drug's generic name is "Lapatinib." This is the patented name of the drug; when the patents expire in seventeen years other manufacturers may make generic forms of the same drug but they will keep the drug label to show the class of generic they are making.

       2) On the other hand, the <u>BRAND NAME</u> of the drug is the name the Pharmaceutical Company gave the drug it manufactures—in our example "Tykerb."

<u>Lapatinib</u> is the ***generic name*** for the drug; <u>Tykerb</u> is the ***brand name*** given by the drug's manufacturer.

Pharmaceutical patents usually provide drug competition protection for seventeen years. After patents expire, other companies may make the same drug (generics) but will brand it with ***their brand name*** for the drug. Many physicians will tend to talk in terms of the drug generic class (Lapatinib), whereas, laymen tend to talk about the brand name of the drug (Tykerb). [physicians = "simvastatin;" laymen = "Zocor." physicians = "acetaminophen;" laymen = "Tylenol." physicians = "trastuzumab;" laymen = "Herceptin."]

Another aspect of Caregiving that is not talked about very much relates to the *CONFIDENCE* your loved one needs to have **in you** as her Caregiver. <u>The Patient has to see her Caregiver as competent and informed</u> before she will place her TRUST in the Caregiver's judgment. If the Caregiver is not informed, the Patient will not "go along" with the Caregiver's choices. By showing the Patient that you have done your homework and can "talk" intelligently with the Oncology Team, you relieve much of your Patient's anxiety or fear about her treatments. Your Patient knows her Caregiver is covering her back and watching out for her wellbeing.

Talk this over with the Oncology Team, so that they understand you, **the caregiver are trying to assume this role and you are in the best position—day in, day out—to do so.** The Family Caregiver is not trying to play Doctor; but the <u>Family Caregiver may be ***the only or best resource***</u> the Oncologist has to follow up on how well the treatment is working with this patient. Ask for their help so you can do a better job.

Most Common Cancer Side Effects

Fatigue:

Cancer related *fatigue* is the most common, and many times the most distressing Side Effect reported by people with cancer. It can come on suddenly and can be overwhelming to the patient. It becomes a steady state in patients with metastasized cancer.

I recall so many discussions of *"I'm tired of being tired."*

My loved one's experience with cancer essentially began with a lumpectomy and chemo, followed by Biotherapy and a five year reprieve of symptoms. Then we discovered that the cancer had metastasized (spread) into the bones of her spine, pelvis, and hips. From that point, the progression seemed to be "two steps forward, one step back." Then it was "two steps forward, two steps back." Then "one step forward, two steps back." And finally, "one-half step forward, three steps back"—as metastasized cancer consumed her body.

Fatigue is usually attributable to multiple factors: beginning with the cancer itself, and the toxicity of the cancer treatments. Also contributing are anemia, nutritional slowdown, sleep dysfunction, and psychological issues like depression, anxiety, chronic pain. Fatigue can be a sign of some other undiagnosed medical condition—for example, heart disease, hypothyroidism, liver or kidney dysfunction, hormonal dysfunction, or anemia.

The list of interventions to lessen cancer related fatigue usually begins with suggestions like, get more rest, conserve energy, try to reduce personal stress, take frequent naps or rest periods, seek assistance with energy consumers like childcare, meal preparation, laundry and house cleaning. Improve nutrition by taking smaller meals more often during the day ["grazing"]. Eat foods rich in protein, vitamins, and iron. Drink plenty of fluids, and for strength, schedule a couple of breaks with consumption of a high protein drink like *Boost* or *Ensu*re. Avoid dizziness or falls by getting up and *moving more slowly, more deliberately*.

Paradoxically, exercise has been shown to improve fatigue. Short walks out in the fresh air, or a mild form of physical therapy might be helpful. It is important to be involved in activities your loved one enjoys, or which relaxes him/her: listening to music, gardening, walking through a park, bird watching, or visiting friends or family.

There is great *courage* involved in combating fatigue and trying to build strength—at a time when your loved one just is "tired of being tired." The emotional toll is huge, and it takes real courage to push forward at the most vulnerable and weak of times. It takes *courage* by both Partners to try to restore QUALITY of LIFE and the normal feeling of WELL-BEING. I think it shows heroic courage by the cancer patient, to dig down into her depths to sustain hope, sustain a positive "can do" attitude, and even to try to sustain humor---evoking a smile in spite of her debilitating weakness.

Nausea and Vomiting:

Although a major concern for individuals undergoing chemotherapy, major strides have been made in the medical control of nausea and vomiting. To control the vomiting, control the nausea. Clearly the toxicity of the chemotherapy can cause nausea. The cancer itself can cause nausea; other medicines like narcotic pain pills (the codines) or antibiotics can cause nausea. Anxiety can also contribute to make nausea worse

In the setting of Infusion therapy, anti-nausea drugs precede the infusion of chemo. Some suggestions to improve the Patient's chances of controlling nausea include: eat lightly before and during chemotherapy; since prevention is the key to control, take an anti-nausea medication before chemotherapy as well as afterwards. Eat "bland foods" like dry toast, crackers, soups, broths, gelatins and other bland foods. Since dehydration can cause nausea, drink plenty of clear liquids, clear juices, tea , 7-Up. Have your Patient rest after meals in an elevated position to help digestion.

If your loved one experiences nausea, report it to the Oncology Team. There are medicines that can help.

Diarrhea:

Perhaps the most embarrassing of the Side Effects, sudden and uncontrolled urges and accidents can completely destroy your loved one's Quality of Life. He/she will not want to do anything, go anywhere, see anyone, for
fear of the suddenness and intensity of the urge and inability to control the elimination.

Diarrhea can be caused by chemotherapy toxins which inflame and irritate the lining of the small intestine or colon. Antibiotics also can cause diarrhea. Bowel infections (e-coli) and tumor growth can cause diarrhea.

Diarrhea can quickly dehydrate the body and deplete minerals (electrolytes) like sodium or potassium which are necessary for tissues to function. Chronic diarrhea can cause serious dehydration which leads to serious health consequences if untreated. Diarrhea associated with chemotherapy or radiation can last a couple of weeks after treatment ends.

<u>CALL your Doctor or Oncologist</u> if your loved one experiences any of the following symptoms:
- high fever (over 101.5 degrees F) for more than 24 hours;
- moderate or severe abdominal pain or cramping;
- blood or undigested food in the diarrhea;
- sudden weight loss (more than about 5 pounds);
- severe diarrhea that shows no improvement over 48 hours;
- diarrhea in persons with serious underlying illnesses for whom the dehydration may have serious consequences: diabetes, heart disease, or HIV

When diarrhea occurs, avoid spicy, rich, fried or greasy foods. Drink 6 to 8 glasses of fluids each day; avoid carbonated or caffeinated beverages, limit milk and milk products. Avoid high fibre grains, bran, wheat products. Avoid citrus juices: orange, pineapple, grapefruit.

Fortunately, there are several over-the-counter remedies for its control like Pepto-Bismol, Immodium AD, and Kaopectate. Consult your loved one's doctor or Oncologist. Keep the rectal area clean and dry; it may experience irritation from the diarrhea.

Diarrhea is ugly—it is messy, it is debilitating, it is depressing. As a Caregiver you may have to address the emotional stress of your loved one as he/she copes with this condition. Be supportive.

Constipation:

Constipation is common gastrointestinal disorder that affects as many as 28% of the North American population; mostly this is from poor nutritional habits, not consuming enough liquids, not consuming enough fibre. Generally, constipation is the infrequent and difficult or painful passage of hard stool.

Because of their cancer and the toxicity of their medications, coupled with poor nutrition and not enough fluids, and frequent inactivity or lack of exercise, constipation is frequent among cancer Patients. Pain medications, chemotherapy, diuretics, and several Biotherapy medications can lead to constipation. Depression, stress, and inactivity can greatly contribute.

Constipation can also be symptomatic of other medical conditions like hemorrhoids, anal fissures, rectal bleeding, or fecal impaction.

The symptoms of constipation in cancer patients include: small hard stools, puffy or bloated abdomen, cramps or stomachache, excessive gas or belching, no bowel movement for more than 3 days, vomiting and nausea, blood in the anal area or in the stool.

Chronic constipation is a real medical condition. Begin by checking diet. It is important to have enough bulk in your loved one's diet to stimulate the bowels. This may be very hard to accomplish, because your loved one is feeling so badly that she does not want to eat, or the food just tastes like sand.

It was always my most difficult challenge to find nutritional foods that would not nauseate her, but would create enough bulk to create stool. It sounds good to say "eat more fiber" but if salads or vegetables or whole grains are just not palatable to your loved one, you may have to resort to soluble fibers like Metamucil.

Further, it is important that enough fluid be consumed to help keep the stool soft. Your Partner should drink at least 6 to 8 glasses of fluids per day. Easy to say—hard to do unless you can develop *a SCHEDULE* for systematically drinking fluids.

Maintain activity. Exercise helps stimulate digestion and prevent constipation. Walking is a great exercise that your loved one may tolerate well; to motivate your Patient, you may need to accompany him/her on short walks around the neighborhood or area.

Over-the-counter medications like Colace, Metamucil, Mylanta, or Senekot may be recommended. Stool softeners may help, especially those coupled with mild laxatives. Your loved one may need regularity laxative protocol if constipation becomes chronic, or if chemotherapy or pain medications are taken in regular doses.   DO NOT use enemas or suppositories if your loved one has a low white blood cells count.

CALL your health care provider if you notice your loved one has not moved her bowels in 3 days, if she complains of an uncomfortable bloated belly, exhibits cramps or vomiting or notices blood in the anal area or stool. Your health care provider may refer you to a Gastroenterologist for further testing.

Peripheral Neuropathy: (nerve irritation in hands or feet)

Neuropathy or nerve irritation or nerve damage can occur in the sensory nerves of the hands or fingers, or feet and toes. Early symptoms include **_tingling_** and/or **_numbness_** in the fingers or toes. Later symptoms might include burning or shooting pains, loss of feeling, extreme sensitivity when touched, and loss of feeling of the affected body part.

In daily life, neuropathy can make it difficult to write or type, open or close zippers, button clothing, pick up objects.....etc. Loss of feeling or sensation **_increases your loved one's risk of injuries or burns_**.

Your loved one may experience a lack of coordination or feelings of weakness. She may drop objects or trip more easily. Motor nerve damage increases the likelihood of falls and accidents.

Nerve damage can be a side effect of certain cancers, and can also be caused by swelling pressure on the nerves from a tumor. And, of course, neuropathy can be a common side effect of certain chemotherapies.

Your loved one's Oncologist will carefully explain the risks of any agents that he feels are necessary to prescribe. Take notes and look up the drugs on MedicineNet.com or WebMD.com. Early detection is always your loved one's best option, so monitor her for any early appearance of symptoms, which may signal the need for modification of her cancer treatments.

Mouth Care during Cancer Treatments:

It is common for cancer patients to develop mouth sores during treatment: chemotherapy, radiation, or biotherapy. It is important to monitor your loved one's mouth if she is undergoing any of the above treatments. Teeth should be brushed by a soft toothbrush after meals and at bedtime. Have your loved one examine her mouth for **redness**, **sores**, or **white patches** inside the mouth or on the tongue. If you notice any of the above, you should inform your Oncologist or Radiologist, and treatment may need to be suspended or modified.

You may want to have your loved one eat small but frequent amounts to limit irritation. We called it "grazing." It may be useful to drink fluids through a straw to bypass irritated areas. You might try to cook foods until tender in texture, or moisten dry foods with mild gravy or sauces.

CALL your Oncologist or Radiologist if you notice problems your loved one is having eating, chewing, or swallowing, or if he/she complains of mouth or throat pain. Get a consultation. Get suggestions. Do not let this condition get out of hand.

The above are the COMMON SIDE EFFECTS experienced by cancer patients during their treatments:

- Fatigue
- Nausea, vomiting
- Diarrhea
- Constipation
- Peripheral Neuropathy
- Mouth sores

Now you as a Caregiver must have ***a new sense of the importance and complexity*** of the Caregiver's home medical role.

In addition to becoming an expert in the above common side effects, each *chemotherapy* cocktail, or *biotherapy* drug, or *radiation* regimen will add additional ***specific side effects*** that you as Caregiver need to know and watch for in order to help the Oncology Team provide your loved one with the best targeted, patient-centered, holistic care that you know she deserves.

Remember, it's all about your Partner, your loved one. .

This is a sacred Trust. Good luck to you and to your loved one for this phase of your journey together.

———————————————————

8)   Medical Records

We have already touched on one aspect of this topic—the *Patient's Medical History*—[See Exhibit 1]. The Medical Records of your Patient *BELONG TO THE PATIENT.*   Copies of medical records may be obtained by request from the Medical Records office of the medical facility where services were performed.   This issue is addressed in the *Patient's Bill of Rights* of the providing institution.   You may also wish to inquire about the institution's Privacy Policy about disclosure of medical records.

Some reasonable time delays may be in effect, allowing the administrative entity to compile the requested Reports. Check with each institution for their administrative policies on obtaining your Patient's medical records.

It is important to keep a file or binder with the medical records incurred by your Patient.

A good plan would be to file all MEDICAL REPORTS (X-ray reports, imaging reports, blood draws, ...etc) in one folder, and create a second folder for FINANCIAL RECORDS .

I would really recommend filing your *Explanations of Benefits* reports from your insurance carrier.   Three-hole punch them and file them into a three ring binder, by date you received them. You can track expenditures, make sure your Deductible and Out-of-Pocket maximum reflect real services received.   Check when they have been met.

This type of record keeping is great when you need to compile your documentation for Income Tax purposes.

[See **Section 17** for a full discussion of *Explanation of Benefits*.]

---

9) <u>**Legal Issues: Advance Directives, Living Will, Power of Attorney:**</u>

Federal and State law delineate the requirement for "Advanced Directives" meaning that the law protects patient rights to make medical decisions affecting them, including the right to accept or refuse medical treatment. In any Emergency, your consent to resuscitation, medical care and treatment is assumed.
This applies to all adult patients regardless of their medical condition.

A *Living Will* is a document signed by the Patient telling any physician NOT to use artificial life support measures if the Patient becomes <u>terminally ill</u>, which means incurably or irreversibly ill, and the administration of life sustaining procedures will only serve to postpone the Patient's death. Life sustaining procedures may include tube feeding or prolonged tubing for artificial respiration. In Colorado, a *Living Will* does not go into effect until two physicians agree in writing that the Patient's condition is terminal.
A *Living Will* also requires the signature of two witnesses, who must not be patients or employees of the facility, creditors, or anyone who may become an inheritor.   It is optional to notarize the document. Legal assistance is not required to complete the document.   A *Living Will* can be changed or canceled at any time.
Of course, if it is changed or canceled, your physician, family, or anyone with a copy should be notified.

[*Living Will*: see **Exhibit 6**]

A *Medical Durable Power of Attorney* is a document signed by your Patient designating an "agent." The agent "stands in" for the Patient when it becomes time to make any or all medical decisions with a doctor.
A *Medical Durable Power of Attorney* can cover more medical decisions than a *Living Will* and is not limited to terminal illness. It may become effective immediately or later when the Patient becomes unable to make medical decisions. <u>Anyone</u> can be appointed the Agent, as long as they are 18 years old, mentally competent, and willing to be the Agent.   If the Spouse is appointed Agent, and the marriage situation changes through divorce, separation or annulment, the Spouse is automatically removed as Agent.   The *Medical Durable Power of Attorney* can be canceled (revoked) at any time.

[*Durable Power of Attorney*: see **Exhibit 7**]

[These forms were developed by the Colorado Advance Directives Consortium (CADC). To obtain complimentary copies of each form, go to www.coloradoadvanceddirectives.com , click on Links and Resources.]

36

IMPORTANT: **Understand that the Patient DOES NOT NEED to have Advance Directives in place BEFORE the Patient can be admitted to a facility or receive care or treatment.** The Patient is required to be _informed_ about these documents at the time of Admission, but because these documents are so personal and so important, it simply makes sense to discuss these issues and prepare the documentation while your loved one is not too ill to think or communicate clearly. Your Patient should be able to tell you what his/her wishes are with regard to medical care. It's all about your loved one. This is a part of your Trust with your loved one.

10) **Medical Devices to Aid Mobility**:

Wheel Chair:

This seems a no-brainer.   Wheel Chairs are very common and quite easy to use. What is not intuitive is that wheel chairs can be very dangerous as the cancer patient loses ambulatory motor skills, or the ability to sit up or stand on her own without your help.

I have learned that the keys to safe use of a wheel chair are (1) Put on the Brakes, and (2) Put on the Brakes, and (3) Check to see if the Brakes are on and holding. *One cannot say it enough*: any time anyone gets into or out of a wheel chair, Put on the Brakes.

I regret to think your experience with your loved one can some day follow a scenario like one I experienced early on. It went something like

> " To pick up your Patient position the wheel chair next to car with car door open...
> Pivot your Patient's legs to dangle outside the car door. Lift your Patient
> to a standing position, (and then you look around and the wheel chair has
> slowly backed toward the rear of the car.") .   Put on the Brakes. One
> experience like this will burn this rule into your mind. Put on the Brakes!"

The second thing I learned is that when you are transferring your Patient from a bed or couch onto the wheel chair, be sure your loved one is wearing shoes, or slippers, or hospital socks— anything with rubber or non-slip soles to keep her from sliding under the chair.

If you are using the wheel chair to move from toilet to vanity, you can easily swing away the foot rests, but if your loved one is going to stand or lean over the vanity to spit after brushing her teeth, put on the brakes, so her legs do not push back the wheel chair as she stands.

38

As your loved one loses the ability to stand on her own, or is weak or unsteady, you may want to obtain a "Transfer Belt" or "Gait Belt" to help you lift her to a standing position, or transfer her from bed to wheel chair, to toilet, to automobile.....etc. This device is a soft belt that goes around your loved one's waist, so you can grab the belt and pull her into you as you lift her to a standing position.

Home Care personnel can assist you to obtain this device. You can also ask your Oncology Social Worker for help. Practice it before you use it.

If she is sitting (as on a couch or side of the bed) dangling her legs over the edge, I found it easier if she would lean forward, putting her "Nose over Toes." By pulling her into yourself, you rotate her forward and upward, and physics principles shift her center of gravity into a standing position. You will not lose your balance because as she stands, her center of gravity will move away from you into her centerline. Try it. "Nose over Toes."

Walker:

A "Walker" is a tube framed device to assist someone who has the strength to stand on their own, but may be unsteady or feel weakness. The handgrips of the walker should be about level with your patient's hips. The patient grasps the walker firmly, lifts it and places it squarely in front of themselves about a foot in front of their body. The rubber tips of the walker should rest firmly on the floor. The person then steps "into the walker" one foot at a time. Then the process is repeated. The frame may be "rested" against for support.

Check the rubber tips. Make sure they are not cracked or missing. Rubber tips can be purchased at most hardware stores if replacement is warranted.

Walkers sometimes have wheels on the front legs. My experience with these is that the wheels make the walker less stable and heavier. I would recommend wheeled walkers only for patients who are **experienced** with walkers, or are no longer able to lift the lighter walkers.

Of course, the real danger with walkers is **throw rugs** which can slip or bunch up when they are hit by the walker front legs. If mobility becomes an issue for your loved one, it is a pretty good strategy to get rid of all throw rugs in the house.

_____

Alignment:

As your loved one gets up and down, bed to wheel chair, to toilet, to TV couch, it is important that you make sure she ends up comfortable in each position.

After you help her lay down on the bed, or on the couch, or sit propped up with pillows, RUN an IMAGINARY LINE in your mind, from head to toe along her body's centerline. <u>Do not leave her alone until this centerline is straight</u>. Otherwise, she will experience stiffness, aching or cramping from being in a strained position.

Centerline alignment, and making sure her bedclothes are not bunched up behind her, will give her <u>more chance to be comfortable</u> for longer periods of time.

Bed-Side Commode:

When mobility deteriorates, the wheel chair run to the bathroom takes more and more time. It is convenient to obtain a bed-side Commode for your loved one. Placed beside the bed, it seems easy to have your loved one sit up, dangle her legs over the side of the bed (slippers or shoes on), ease her into a standing position, pivot her, and sit her down on the Commode. Reverse the steps to get her back into bed.

What I learned that I was not prepared for, was even though the Commode is stable with four legs grounded to the floor, the Toilet Lid of the Commode leans back against a low pipe running along the back. An OPEN toilet lid on a Commode CAN NOT SUSTAIN MUCH WEIGHT, should your loved one lean back against it.
And this can happen if she is groggy from pain medication or anxiety medication.

This lid is not like a toilet lid that leans back against the water tank behind the toilet.

Be vigilant <u>that your loved one does NOT LEAN BACK against the open commode lid.</u> It will not support her weight. And you will be dealing with not only a messy spill on the floor, but your loved one can easily fall and break a bone or at least receive serious bruising.

Hand Rails:

Of course, this discussion depends upon the level of ambulatory (walking) mobility your loved one still has. Yet, it really does not matter; this is a safety issue even the most mobile and athletic can find some benefit from. Hand rails on stairs in the home are required by building codes in most jurisdictions in the United States. Let's assume they are installed and go into the bathroom.

I believe it is necessary to install hand rails around the bath tub, or upon entrance to the shower. For one thing, hand rails just makes getting in or out easier. They also help make getting up or down easier. And finally, they frequently ***prevent falls***.

I have heard one person complain that handrails may make the bathroom appear more "institutional." Before rebutting the person who said this, I thought to myself, "hey, you can hang face towels or bath towels from them and you will not even notice them." Then I thought that I have read that in the home, ***most falls occur in the bathroom, don't they?***

I guess this comes down to personal preference. But if I can prevent even one fall in the bathtub for my loved one, there is no question here. The hand rails were installed. And I really DO NOT think they make the bathroom look "institutional." *They show concern, and caring*.

Pocket Doors:

Another personal preference. When my loved one lost ambulatory mobility, she was dependent upon assistance to get to the bathroom and around the house, and we relied upon her wheel chair or her walker.

I noticed the layout of the bathroom: the vanity on the left, bath tub/shower directly ahead, and toilet to the right end of the room. The door into the bathroom opened into the middle of the room, and would swing 180 degrees to the right against the wall to the side of the toilet. But if the door was left partially open, ***it required her to maneuver her wheel chair around the door*** to reach the toilet.

Pocket Doors were the answer. Pocket doors slide in and out, from inside the wall. When open they just disappear into the wall   They close and even lock; they provide complete privacy equivalent to a normal swinging door. A good carpenter can install them by removing one side of the drywall, installing the pocket door, then replacing and refinishing the drywall. All that is left is painting to match the rest of the wall.

We installed pocket doors into all bathrooms in the house. **What a convenience!**

```
┌─────────────────────────────────────────┐
│                                           │
│           INSURANCE MANAGEMENT            │
│                                           │
└─────────────────────────────────────────┘
```

A recent study by the Harvard Medical School concludes that in 2007, **62.1% of all bankruptcies in America were attributed to the** *high cost* of medical care—up from about 50% in 2001.
Of the number who filed bankruptcy in 2007, ***almost 80% had health insurance***.

A follow-up telephone survey done in five States suggests ***that in 2009, after the meltdown of the economy, the number of bankruptcies citing medical causes may be as high as 68%.***

Extrapolate to today **70%? 74%?**

And it has been recently reported [09/2010] , ***that the number of medically uninsured Americans has gone up from 44 million to 51 million.***

What this data suggests is

1) Health Care Reform is **even more important today** than it was in 2009 when it was passed;

2) Definite ***fine tuning*** needs to be continued to make the new Health Care Reform Act become more functionally useful and financially accurate---even exceeding the Health Care Reform legislation enacted in 2009; and

3) if 80% of the 2007 bankruptcy filers *had medical insurance* , they must have had the **wrong insurance** for their needs.

I have included the following article from the *Washington Post* in summary form to corroborate the above data:

The Washington Post reported:

New Study: Bankruptcy Tied To Medical Bills

By Sarah Lovenheim

Sixty-two percent of all bankruptcies filed in 2007 were linked to medical expenses, according to a nationwide study released today by the American Journal of Medicine. That's nearly 20 percentage points higher than that pool of respondents reported were connected to medical costs in 2001.

Of those who filed for bankruptcy in 2007, nearly 80 percent had health insurance. Respondents who reported having insurance indicated average expenses of just under $18,000. Respondents who filed and lacked insurance had average medical bills of nearly $27,000.

Since 2007, the number of Americans without insurance has increased, and filing for bankruptcy has become more difficult due to more stringent laws, according to the report.

> "Out-of-pocket medical costs averaged $17,943. for all medically bankrupt families: $26,971. for uninsured patients, $17,749. for those with private insurance at the outset, $14,633. for those with Medicaid, $12,021. for those with Medicare, and $6545 for those with VA/military coverage.
>
> Among common diagnoses, nonstroke neurologic illnesses such as Multiple Sclerosis were associated with the highest out-of-pocket expenditures (mean $34,167), followed by diabetes($26,971), injuries ($25,096), ..and heart disease ($21,955)."

[Source: *American Journal of Medicine,* reported in The Washington Post, (06/04/2009)]

Selected costs of some of the most commonly prescribed cancer drugs:

GlaxoSmithKline's *Tykerb* (hormonal signal inhibitor of HER-2 receptors responsible for certain high-risk cancers in women, decrease tumor-causing breast cancer stem cells) = ($4,737./ month).
Genentech's *Herceptin* [IV breast cancer inhibitor of HER2 cancer receptors] = ($3,945./6wk intervals).
Novartis' *Gleevec* [myeloid leukemia cancer of white blood cells] = ($4,500./ month)
Genentech's *Avastin*, [colon/colorectal, lung cancers, cuts blood vessel supply to tumor] = ($2,898./month for its lowest dosage.)
Celgene's *Revlimid*, [breast, lung, pancreatic some lymphoma cancers; maintenance therapy = ($10,806. per month).
Dendreon's *Provenge* (one-time targeted treatment for terminal prostate cancer, approved April, 2010 = ($93,000). [I was surprised to read that with regard to Provenge, the M.D.Anderson Cancer Center (Houston, TX) is considering a lottery to pick 2 patients per month from the 150 eligible patients; two a month is all they can handle. Stem cells must be removed and a specifically targeted chemo concoction is mixed with the cells for infusion back into the patient.]
Stem cell transplants for other cancers run upwards of $78,000. just for the procedure.

[Sources: *Clinical Pharmacology*, Assoc. Press, DenverPost.com 9/27/10, and pharmacychecker.com.]

Real Life Personal Example-----Cancer Treatments are very expensive:

Explanation of Benefits statements describe medical billing for services provided, along with date of the service, as well as "adjusted" medical service payments by the insurer. We kept a three ring binder with each *Explanation of Benefits* statement we received from our own Insurance carrier. I would scan it for any line item that would be surprising or confusing; I would sum all the totals at the end of the year.

Totaling all my wife's 2009 medical expenditures:

[Office Visits, chemo, fluids, imaging...]

Medical Provider Services
Billed to Insurance carrier
$ 197,725.00

From our cash flow: the medical insurance monthly premium I paid for my loved one was **$292.00** per month (times 12 months = **$3,504.00** for the year)--- plus her Insurance Plan carried an **Out-of-Pocket Maximum = $5,800.00** Our personal *Payout total* for the year = **$9,304.00**

[I paid $ 9,304.00 for her insurance for the year; she received $197,725.00 worth of care. If we had selected conventional insurance coverage, we would have had the standard "80:20" insurance—{the insurance carrier pays 80% and the patient pays 20% after deductible.). Twenty percent of $197,725. = just under $40,000. This was for 2009. *Each of the last four years after her metastasis* was about the same! We had no options for raising this amount of resources, even selling our house.]

This is **why** you **must** consider Insurance Plans with **"Out-of-Pocket " Maximums!** Almost every commercial insurer provides at least one plan option that offers an out of pocket maximum for the consumer.

11) Choosing the Right Insurance Plan:

Find out if the Cancer Patient is eligible for membership in a GROUP INSURANCE PLAN:

1) Group Plans cost less; their *premiums are discounted* relative to the number of subscribers;

2) Many Group Plans also provide individuals with *a partial subsidy* of their premiums;

3) Most Group Plans *waive the "pre-existing medical condition" exclusion* from coverage.

Find out if the Cancer care facility used by your Cancer Patient is IN-NETWORK of the list of contracted medical entities defined by your Insurance carrier as within the approved network; or find out if it is an OUT-OF-NETWORK facility. The expenses paid by the Cancer Patient are going to cost *twice as much* for Out-of-Network care as for In-Network care. This is one of the ways Insurance carriers contain costs; remember, they define their discounts with In-Network providers.

Find out whether or not PRESCRIPTION DRUGS are covered by the Plan you are researching. Plans differ as to whether or not prescription drugs are included; some make you purchase a supplemental Prescription Drug Plan. This is especially true in the case of some Medicare Advantage plans.

If the Patient is in a *maintenance mode* with regard to her disease, PRESCRIPTION DRUGS MAY BE THE LARGEST EXPENDITURE you will need to make in the upcoming Plan Year. Do not overlook this matter; once you elect to go with a certain insurance plan, you may not be able to change your mind or add in a Prescription Drug supplement for the remainder of the year.

Decision Rule: Check to see how PRESCRIPTION DRUGS are covered by the Plans you are researching.

----

12) KEY PROVISION OF INSURANCE PLANS FOR CANCER PATIENTS:

Insurance Plans are required by law to follow a template outline of their provisions, so those searching for insurance coverage have information that is **comparable across Plans**. The following is from the general **Outline of Benefits** from the first section of her actual Medical Insurance Policy:

Part A: Type of Coverage

1) Type of Plan   (HMO, PPO, PPPS, ...etc)
2) Out-of-Network Care covered?   (Yes)
3) Areas where Plan is Available   (International)

Part B: Summary of Benefits

4) Annual Deductible (for individual coverage, for family coverage)

5) OUT-OF-POCKET MAXIMUM   (for individual coverage, for family coverage, and whether or not the Deductible is included in the Plan's Out-of-Pocket Maximum).

6) Lifetime Benefit Maximum (this will be dropped in 2014 under new *Health Care Reform Act* legislative rules.)

............etc.

Decision Rule: Look for Plans that provide an **_OUT-OF-POCKET MAXIMUM_** for the Cancer Patient and her Partner to consider.

 Begin with plans for Individuals, and then consider plans for Families. We elected individual plans, because they provided us a more financially feasible option--a lower out-of-pocket than family plans; our best option was for separate individual plans from different insurance carriers.

Out-of-Pocket Maximums can be found in all types of insurance coverage: HMOs, PPOs, PFFS, HDHP, and Catastrophic insurance plans.

Perhaps the ***most encouraging*** aspect of the new Health Care Reform legislation is the fact that Congress has voted to eliminate the double standard that exists today, where Members of Congress have access to exceptional medical coverage.

In 2014 when the Health Care Reform Bill becomes fully operable, Members of Congress will no longer have privileged access to their own Federal Insurance Plan, and will have to find and purchase their medical insurance through the State insurance exchanges that start in 2014, just like all other Americans. The insurance exchanges will be mainly for those who do not have Employer provided insurance, and will offer options closely resembling those that all 8 million Federal Workers have today.

An AARP Bulletin, ***Special Report,*** issued in May, 2010, shows that Congress has elected to protect its basic coverage and continue the Out-of-Pocket provision they currently enjoy. A summary of the ***Special Report*** appears on the following page.

[For a list of the Medicare Insurance Plans with an Out-of-Pocket Maximum, visit **Exhibit 8**.]

Similar Plans are usually **also available** from the same insurance companies for those who are not yet qualified for Medicare because of age, or Plan availability. CALL the insurance companies you have an interest in, or consult your Oncology Social Worker for advice.

A new option becoming available is that some Pharmaceutical companies may provide some limited financial assistance, up to the Out-of-Pocket maximum of the Patient's insurance, if their drug is prescribed for treatment. Call your treatment drug Pharmaceutical manufacturer to see if this is an option they provide.

[Visit: *NeulastaFirstStep.com* from Amgen].

To find help to pay for Medicines, this list was provided by the Denver Post: visit:

Novartis:	www.patientassistancenow.com
Patient Advocate Foundation:	www.patientadvocate.org or www.copays.org
CancerCare:	www.cancercare-copay.org
Chronic Disease Fund:	www.cdfund.org

What about Health Care Reform? [Note: Out-of-Pocket Max retained}

AS GOOD AS CONGRESS

Many Americans will get the same deal as members of Congress. The new law requires legislators to purchase coverage through State insurance exchanges, that start in 2014. Benefit options will mirror options held by Federal workers today.

Coverage Provisions	Federal Health Benefits today	New Health Care Reform Law
Choice of Insurance plans?	Plans of all types, available through national insurance exchange, for employees. dependents, retirees .	Plans of all types, available through employer or public coverage
Benefits?	Variable, but with specific minimum benefit package.	Variable, but with specific minimum benefit package.
Higher rates based on health?	No	No
Higher rates based on gender?	No	No
Subsidies?	Yes, up to 75% of premiums	Yes, reduced premiums based on income
Out of Pocket Maximum?	Yes	Yes
Dependent children?	Yes, through age 21	Yes, through age 25
Year round Prescription Drugs?	Yes	Yes, narrows/eliminates Medicare Part D "doughnut hole"-2020
Plans must meet standards?	Yes	Yes
Plans posted online?	Yes	Yes
Denial for health status, or pre- existing conditions?	No	No
Switch Plans each year?	Yes	Yes
Abortion coverage?	Only rape / incest, or endanger the woman's life	Only rape / incest, or endanger the woman's life. If she receives federal subsidies insurers who cover abortion may charge additional premiums.
Coverage of Illegal immigrants?	Not applicable	Specifically prohibited

[Source: AARP: www.aarp.org/health/health-care-reform/info-04-2010/]

13) **High Deductible Health Plans:**

If you currently have medical insurance (including Medicare) which pays 80% , **leaving the Patient to cover the 20% balance on each bill,** cancer will bankrupt you—First you can count on burning your way through your savings, then burning through your 401-K retirement savings, and finally burning through the equity you have built up in your home.   Medicare, by itself will do this, because the Patient must make up the 20% part of costs.   Let's look at a Medicare example:

Imagine, if you expect cancer expenses that will exceed $30,000.00 in the insurance Plan Year, [and this amount will barely cover a four month chemotherapy treatment protocol.]   Medicare will pay 80%, but YOU will be responsible for at least $6,000.00 [or 20%] out-of-pocket.. That amount ($6,000.) *exceeds* a High Deductible Health Plan's *Out-of-Pocket Maximum* found in many private insurance plans.

Decision Rule: **Patient or Caregiver should consider HIGH DEDUCTIBLE Health Plans (HDHP).**

[Mandated by Congress, these Plans have less expensive premiums than most insurance plans, These Plans require the Insured Patient to pay the "high deductible" UP FRONT, before any benefits are paid out by the Plan. But, these Plans have a mandated Out-Of-Pocket Maximum which *includes* the "high deductible" amount in its calculation.]

Another Example:

For the Plan year 2010, *Anthem Blue Cross/ Blue Shield* provides an HDHP Plan with a "High Deductible" of **$3,500.** for individual coverage, which **must be paid up front** *before* the Plan pays any benefits.   The "high" deductible is $3,500, compared to the "normal" deductible of $1,500.

But, the Plan also has an Out-of-Pocket maximum of **$5,950.** for individual coverage, *AND* the **$3,500.** High Deductible is **included** in the Out-of-Pocket Maximum amount.

As a Cancer Caregiver, I have learned that we would meet the Out-of-Pocket Maximum for my spouse **in February or March** of each Plan Year. *The Plan then covered all expenses— prescription drugs, medical procedures and treatments, physician visits, chemotherapy—for the remainder of the Plan Year.*

A final consideration for HDHP plans is that they also come with a mandated **Health Savings Account [HSA].** The idea of a Health Savings Account is that pre-tax funds can be deposited into the HSA, and subsequently paid out *tax free* for medical expenses incurred by the Patient (HSA account owner). Payments from an HSA are made by check, with patient or joint owner signatures.

This is a *huge incentive* to save for future medical expenses. and to save on income taxes from the funds deposited. There is an annual limit to how much can be deposited each year. Any major banking institution can describe the eligibility requirements and deposit requirements for the HSA. And disbursements from the HSA are *TAX FREE*.

Medicaid

Colorado Medicaid is a public health insurance program for families, children and pregnant women, persons who are blind, or persons with disabilities, and the elderly—who are low income Colorado residents having very limited assets and resources.

Colorado Medicaid programs are administered through the **Department of Health Care Policy and Financing,** and all programs offered are listed on their website:

www.colorado.gov/HCPF

You may also want to visit the U.S. Dept of Health and Human Services, Centers for Medicare and Medicaid Services (CMS) which describes the Federal side of Medicaid and the enabling policies:

www.CMS.gov

The Regular Medicaid program allows Medicaid clients to get medical services **from any Provider** who accepts Medicaid clients; there is no need to get referrals for care. Physicians are not required to take on any new patients. Copayments are also required for most services.

Many groups of people are covered by Medicaid—those over 65, pregnant women, children, blind or disabled.

Even within these groups, though, certain requirements must be met. These may include your age, whether you are pregnant, disabled, blind, or aged; your income and resources (like bank accounts, real property, or other items that can be sold for cash); and whether you are a U.S. citizen or a lawfully admitted immigrant. The rules for counting your income and resources vary from state to state and from group to group. There are special rules for those who live in nursing homes and for disabled children living at home.

Other Programs administered by the Colorado <u>Department of Health Care Policy and Financing</u> that may have some relevance for cancer patients might include:

- Medicaid
- Child Health Plan Plus
- Breast and Cervical Cancer Program
- Non-Emergency Medical Transportation

There are differing *income* limitations for each of these programs, as well as *asset* and *resource*s limitations. In general, rates are tied to the **Federal Poverty Levels** attached as **<u>Exhibit 5</u>**. *Asset and resource limits* run around $2,000. for individuals, and $3,000. for families.

In general, you should apply for Medicaid if you have limited income and resources. You must match one of the descriptions above: over 65, or woman, or pregnancy, or child, or blind, or disabled. . Even if you are not sure whether you qualify, if you or someone in your family **needs** health care, you can apply for Medicaid and have a qualified case worker evaluate your situation.

Another twist under the new Health Care law, are the following reforms which took effect <u>Sept. 23, 2010</u>:

- Young adults can return/remain to their families' health care coverage until their 26th birthday;
- Plans can no longer cancel coverage if you become sick;
- Plans can no longer set lifetime dollar limits on coverage; if you were canceled because you reached your Plan's limit, you will be able to rejoin the Plan.
- Limits on annual medical expenses will be phased out over 3 years;
- Plans in existence on Mar 23, 2010 will receive "grandfathered" status, protected so Americans who are satisfied with their policies can keep them.

[Source: AARP Bulletin: <u>AARP.org/health</u>]

The option to have a "medically needy" program allows the States to extend Medicaid eligibility to additional qualified persons <u>who may have too much income</u> to qualify under the mandatory needy groups. This option allows them to "spend down" to Medicaid eligibility by incurring medical and/or remedial care expenses to offset their excess income, thereby reducing it to a level below the maximum allowed by that State's Medicaid plan.

[Source: www.<u>CMS.gov</u>]

For more information, call HealthColorado, the Medicaid insurance enrollment broker, at 303-839-2120 (metro Denver) or 1-888-367-6557 (outside metro Denver)

---

14) OTHER RESOURCES for THOSE WHO DO NOT HAVE INSURANCE:

The previous discussion *presumes* that the people involved in the Caregiver and Patient Partnership have insurance to work with in managing their condition.

 IF THE PATIENT DOES NOT HAVE INSURANCE, they should immediately consult the Social Workers involved in the Clinic or Hospital or the Oncologists who can make recommendations that might be pursued to obtain coverage or assistance.

The American medical system is loathe to turn away patients simply on the basis they cannot pay. Alternative forms of financial support, Foundation assistance, Pharmaceutical assistance, and programs of the National Institute of Health, and the American Cancer Society should be pursued. Religious organizations may be a source of financial support or human services.   Even private funding may be made available under certain circumstances. CONSULT YOUR MEDICAL SOCIAL WORKER OR COUNSELOR FOR INFORMATION.

Let me interject a word of ***caution*** on a new scheme coming into the open to obtain cancer resources:

A new approach for financial support for diagnosed **advanced cancer patients** is coming into *vogue----**purchasing their Life Insurance policy*** for a reduced amount of its cash value. After a diagnosis of a six months life-limiting illness, some companies may approach your loved one with the proposition for a quick cash settlement. They will buy a patient's life insurance policy for a discounted amount of cash, and the patient must sign the insurance policy over to them. When the patient dies, they will collect the full amount of the policy!

RESIST ANY PANIC of struggling to pay medical bills, and looking down the road at the magnitude of proposed cancer costs.   GET ADVICE from a qualified Attorney or Medical Social Worker ***before*** you make any decisions. This cannot be undone once committed. Band Aids do not really heal wounds.

[To obtain more information about these options visit:
<sellyourinsurance.com,> or <lifeinsurancebuyers.com>
BUT be very critical of these "creative" options.]

Getting US Covered

Another option to check by those who do not currently have medical insurance coverage and who have been DENIED COVERAGE BECAUSE OF A PRE-EXISTING MEDICAL CONDITION, might be ***Getting US Covered—a provision of the new Health Care Reform Act*** that went into effect in July, 2010. This program is a bridge to 2014, when comprehensive health reform is fully implemented.

To **qualify** for this health plan, applicants must be Colorado residents and U.S. citizens or lawfully residing in the U.S Applicants must have a <u>pre-existing condition</u> that has prevented them from getting health coverage. Premiums will range from $115.00 per month to $601.00 per month for non smokers, depending upon an individual's age and where she lives. The Plan carries a $2,500.00 deductible and copays of $30 for Primary Care and $45 for Specialist physician visits. Members will pay no more than $5,950.00 in OUT-OF-POCKET costs per year.

Getting US Covered is administered by two non-profit insurance entities—Rocky Mountain Health Plans, and Cover Colorado. ***Getting US Covered*** will phase out in 2014, when insurance companies must offer coverage to everyone, regardless of pre-existing conditions.

[For a full review of options, go to www.covercolorado.org or www.rmhp.org]

Colorado Indigent Care Program [CICP]

The Colorado Indigent Care Program [CICP] provides discounted health care services to low income individuals, at participating providers. McKee Medical Center, Poudre Valley Hospital, Estes Park Medical Center, and the Medical Center of the Rockies are participating providers.

[To find all participating providers, visit <u>colorado.gov/hcpf</u>]

CICP is not a health insurance program. Applicants will be given a "CICP rating" based on income and resources; these ratings will determine the patient's level of copayments at each facility. CICP is funded with Federal and State dollars to partially compensate the participating entities to provide health care to the uninsured, or the underinsured, at or below 250% of the Federal Poverty level. [Covered individuals must not exceed income of $ 2,256.00 per month; a family of 4 must not exceed income of $ 4,594.00 per month.]

However, under CICP clients do not have to pay more than 10% of their income and resources towards copayments in each calendar year. For example a family of four with annual income of $ 16,500.00 will not have to pay more than $ 1,650. Patients must keep receipts to show proof of payments.

Although each Hospital or Clinic decides which services are medically necessary, ***all Hospital providers MUST provide Emergency Care.*** Many also provide Urgent Care and some inpatient care and primary care. Check each facility or your Medical Social Worker for more information. This Program is administered by the Department of Health Care Policy and Financing: colorado.gov/hcpf

---

Medicaid's Breast and Cervical Cancer Program [BCCP]

The Breast and Cervical Cancer Program (BCCP) is a Medicaid program for women who have been diagnosed with breast or cervical cancer at certain screening clinics called Women's Wellness Connection sites (WWC). BCCP also covers breast and cervical conditions that may lead to cancer if not treated.

The initial hurdle to be overcome for eligibility in this program is that the diagnosis must have been made at a specific screening Clinics, called Women's Wellness Connection (WWC) sites. Screenings at the WWC sites is usually *free.* For a list of sites, visit:

[www. cdphe.state.co.us/pp/cwcci/countysites.pdf]

Eligibility qualifications are for WOMEN WHO:

- Have been diagnosed through a WWC site;
- Are between 40 and 64 years old;
- Have an income less than 250% of the Federal Poverty Level;
- Have not had a mammogram or Pap smear test in the last year;
- Do not have health insurance or it does not cover breast or cervical cancer treatment;
- Are not currently enrolled in Medicaid and are not eligible for Medicare; and
- Are U.S. citizens or qualified non-citizens.

To qualify, the patient does not need to be determined disabled, and there are NO INCOME or ASSET LIMITS, and the individual cannot apply directly through Larimer County. The client must apply through the specific Women's Wellness Connection Site of which they are a member and where their screenings took place.

The specific Women's Wellness Connection site will be responsible for assisting interested women in filling out the Application for BCCP benefits through this program. For questions, contact

[Colorado Department of Health Care
Policy and Financing, at 303-866-2385
or diane.stayton@state.co.us.]

[The Cancer Caregiver may also wish to visit
www.Affordable-Health-Insurance-Plans.org
or if your loved one is over 55, you may want to
visit www.benefitscheckup.org]

Foundation Assistance

Each major hospital institution, whether a member of a family of hospitals, or a stand-alone hospital, most likely has its own Hospital Foundation. Hospital Foundations are non-profit entitles engaged in fund raising and maintaining funds for use by the Hospital most often in capital building projects, or as self-insurance against major disasters.

Most of these Hospital Foundations also earmark some portion of the funds at their disposal for patient care. These funds improve access to care and can be dispersed to assist patients who are only able to pay a moderate portion of their care or patients who are uninsured and completely unable to pay any portion of their care.

BEGIN by consulting your Cancer Center MEDICAL SOCIAL WORKER, or PATIENT NAVIGATOR. The Hospital may also employ Financial Counselors within their Patient Billing Offices. This consultation will be handled in a sensitive and confidential manner that respects the privacy and dignity of your loved one, and your family.

A financial evaluation will be conducted to determine eligibility and which financial assistance plan best meets the needs of this patient and his/her family. Eligibility may also pose the requirement that the patient must apply for and be accepted by their State Medicaid. Each Foundation will impose differing eligibility requirements.

[Again, for 2010 *Federal Poverty Levels*, see **Exhibit 5**]

Managing Insurance issues can be almost a full time occupation, given the complexity of the issues and bureaucracy of the systems.   But the financial consequences to the Patient and Caregiver are extreme if this aspect of paying for medical care is ignored or taken for granted. Don't be cavalier about insurance.

15)   Getting a Case Manager within the Insurance Firm:

It is always good idea to have a consumer advocate *WITHIN* the Insurance Firm, who can assist the Patient or Caregiver *to navigate through the complex labyrinth* of bureaucracy of Private Insurance firms.   The firm will provide an RN on payroll who can answer medical and accounting questions, or "work the system" to obtain solutions.

Call the firm and request that a **Case Manager** be assigned to the Patient's account.

---

16)   Insurance Records / EOBs / Claims:

The FINANCIAL aspect of Medical Records involves the EXPLANATION OF BENEFITS [EOB]. The cancer Patient's insurance carrier will periodically or monthly send your Patient an *Explanation of Benefits* paid out for services provided.

These documents are very important for you to determine the *accuracy and completeness of the financial liability* of your cancer Patient.

[I have experienced the shock of receiving an invoice from a hospital for services provided *1.5 years* earlier that they had not billed.   (Do not assume that EOY fiscal years mean automatic closure of the books. Subsequent <u>internal audits</u> revealed the billing error, and so I received the statement.) After much research and correspondence, I ended up finding out that the billed services provided took place on a day where my loved one was receiving cancer treatment at another hospital. Further research of the billing coding revealed that the services that were billed were coded as related to *birthing*—a medical condition not possible for my wife. The billing Hospital backed off on the charges and wrote them off.]

DO NOT ASSUME you are always being billed accurately; check your EOBs, ask questions, do not be afraid to obtain clarification or question vague billing items on your Statements.

The ***Explanation of Benefits*** provides the record of <u>medical services provided and billed</u> to your insurance carrier, as well as the record of <u>Benefits paid</u> by the Patient's medical insurance .

The EOB typically describes the DATE and TYPE of medical service provided, WHICH MEDICAL GROUP or PHYSICIAN provided the service, and a record of CO-INSURANCE and COPAYS made; It also lists HOW MUCH WAS BILLED for the service and HOW MUCH WAS PAID by the insurance company. The EOB may also go so far as to list the amount the ***Patient is responsible to pay***, as well as how much you have paid against your annual DEDUCTIBLE.

[Example *Explanation of Benefits*, See **Exhibit 9**]

Daily business transactions in our lives might lead one to assume that "billed" and "paid" would be the same amount; but in the world of medical insurance this is not the case. The "billed" amount is the full amount the medical entity (hospital, clinic, laboratory...ect) bills to the insurance company. But because of ***discounts contracted*** when the insurance company signed up to provide medical insurance services to the entity, the "billed" amount is ADJUSTED to reflect the discounted amount that was contractually agreed upon, and PAYMENT is rendered for the adjusted amount.

The point is that <u>accounting mistakes are made between all the entities making these adjustments,</u> and these mistakes may not be caught before the cancer Patient is issued an Invoice or Bill for Services.

What does this mean for the Caregiver?

     1) Keep a file or folder listing the Explanation of Benefits [EOB] by your Patient's insurance.   Ideal for these records would be a three-ring binder.

     2) Make payments to medical entities ***only when you can reconcile*** the Invoices received from the different Medical Service Providers (Physician Groups, Laboratories, Clinics,....etc) against the *Explanation of Benefits*.   I sometimes have enclosed duplicate copies of the relevant EOBs to the billing entities as explanations of payment that is less than requested.

Decision Rule: ***ALWAYS LET YOUR PRIMARY INSURANCE WORK FIRST***.
               Then, reconcile back to your Primary Insurance Explanation of Benefits to **identify any additional liability** or further obligations on your part.

----

17) Denials / Challenges:

Keep excellent Medical Records. Contact your Oncologist, and Insurance Case Worker,

Read over the Insurance Plan booklet "Statement of Benefits" to see how Appeals are outlined, and read the steps of the Appeal or Grievance processes.

Particularly annoying are situations where a ***third party*** provides Utilization Management services to the Insurance company.   These are outside or ancillary private companies hired by the Insurance carrier to assess the "medical necessity" of a proposed procedure and advise your Primary Insurance company whether or not to approve it.

This just means that it is harder or more complicated to undo a Denial .

Decision Rule: *ACT*--   do not put this off. Time is of the essence. Deadlines for Appeals ***must*** be met.

HOUSEHOLD CARE MANAGEMENT

TAKING OVER

```
┌─────────────────────────────────────────┐
│                                           │
│       HOUSEHOLD CARE MANAGEMENT           │
│                                           │
│            TAKING OVER                    │
│                                           │
└─────────────────────────────────────────┘
```

18) Cleaning and Maintenance:

Caregiver and loved one should discuss this matter. Caregiver cannot assume it all. This is an easy area to get help, to free up the Caregiver to attend to the Patient. Assistance is available, with varying charges or rates including voluntary free household cleaning from Churches or religious organizations. Check into: family, friends or neighbors, Home Care, Pathways Hospice, your Church, Synagogue or Mosque.

[I recall the difficulty of a couple of instances of Patient care involving necessity for Patient hygiene during the night due to diarrhea; we found these late night needs were *handled best by obtaining household help during the day*, freeing up the Caregiver for night duty.]

Important: get Household help during the daytime, so you as Caregiver can spend more quality time with your loved one, and be better equipped and alert to handle your loved one's calls for help during the night.

> [Check: www.cleaningforareason.org for once a month free home cleaning for women undergoing chemotherapy. Funded by the Susan G. Komans Foundation.]

19) Paying Bills / Managing the Money:

Organize these functions. Schedule the same times of month to pay the bills and stick to it. Do not let medical necessities crowd out these important financial maintenance functions. You can pay bills while your loved one is undergoing infusion treatment, if necessary.

In advanced stages of cancer, you may do some *"what if...?"* household financial worksheets. If your loved one is a contributor to the family living expenses, run a spreadsheet calculation of what it would look like if her portion of the household budget were suddenly no longer available. The paradox is *live in the moment one day at a time with your loved one, but plan ahead so you will be prepared to live in the future moment.*

Do not neglect to make timely payments on your mortgage and your medical insurance; these are two matters you certainly do not want to let lapse or lose.

20) Nutrition Management:

Your Oncologist is concerned about Patient *STRENGTH, and ABILITY TO TOLERATE* toxic chemo medications.   Dosing and Duration decisions depend upon Patient strength. Consequently, it becomes important to focus meal preparation and nutritional value on building and maintaining Patient strength. It is useful to keep records of nutrition intake for discussion with Oncological Team.

[My loved one would say she had eaten "a bowl of oatmeal" when she really only tasted two tablespoons of oatmeal in the morning--clearly not enough for building strength. I began to keep a *Nutrition Log*, for documentation and for future discussions with our Oncology Team.]

[For *Nutrition Log* form: See **Exhibit 10**]

 In addition, it is important to keep in mind that the ***portions*** the Patient can tolerate may become much smaller and smaller as the disease progresses.   But the need for Patient STRENGTH increases.   Consequently, it is important to *become more creative* in preparing meals with high nutritional value, and to monitor the protein intake (for energy) of each meal. It is usually more successful to have the Patient consume ***many small meals,*** [grazing] rather than two or three standard meals. It is also useful to work in ***high protein drinks*** like ***Boost*** or ***Ensure*** into the daily regimen either with meals or as in-between drinks.   Separate sheets may be needed to record **fluid** intake.

Most Useful Nutrition resources:

- National Cancer Inst. booklet on *Eating Hints for CancerPatients*

- Sanofi-Aventis booklet on *Eating Well Through Cancer*

- American Cancer Society booklet *Nutrition for the Person with Cancer during Treatment*; especially, the comprehensive and informative Section on "Managing Eating Problems during Treatment."

For a complementary approach to the matters of nutrition you may want to explore the site www.nutritionfacts.org which lists numerous studies of the positive effects from selected foods or herbal supplements on cancer or on the body's immune system.

I recognize the importance of balanced nutrition, and I have familiarity with the food groups which balanced food intake with exercise—*MyPyramid*.   However, as the disease progresses and your loved one undergoes cancer treatments, or is in pain, anxiety or stress, appetite may shrink to actual revulsion for food. "It tastes like eating sand."   Simplify to basic simple foods, and consult your cancer Dietitian for help. This is a critically important issue because your patient's *physical* strength must be supported if she is going to tolerate the toxicities of her treatments.

21) Physical Therapy / Flexibility / Range of Motion: :

Because of the fundamental importance of STRENGTH for Patient survival and tolerance of increasingly toxic medications, your loved one might want to explore options for physical therapy: either a home workout station, or a mild workout program like that at the Rocky Mountain Cancer Rehabilitation Institute [RMCRI] at the University of Northern Colorado in Greeley.

Any holistic approach to the treatment of cancer will integrate programs of Cancer Physical Rehabilitation into their regimens of treatments. One example I found useful is the video on cancer rehabilitation that was produced by Cancer Treatment Centers of America. This video explains the holistic philosophy of inclusion of physical rehabilitation into cancer treatment.

[See: www.cancercenter.com]

```
┌─────────────────────────────────┐
│     HOUSEHOLD MANAGEMENT         │
│                                  │
│     PERSONAL HOME CARE           │
└─────────────────────────────────┘
```

22) PERSONAL CARE / MODESTY / INTIMACY:

Personal Issue of Hair Loss:

If *Fatigue* is the most commonly reported side effect of cancer treatments, one of the most devastating can be ***hair loss***.

Women often associate beauty, femininity, and identity with their hair. When female hair loss occurs, it can seem, at first, to threaten your loved one. Fear, intimidation, and a lack of self confidence often accompanies hair loss. With the thought that your loved one is losing her beauty and the physical trait that makes her special as a woman, your loved one may even become depressed and dismayed at thinking about what hair loss may mean for her future.

Cancer Chemotherapy treatments are designed to attack fast growing cells. Hair is usually one of the first casualties of chemo. But Medical Oncology Clinicians seem to me less concerned about hair loss than their patients, because they know and have experienced hair regrowth and replacement most usually occurring two to four months after treatments are discontinued. Scalp hair may come back a little "kinkier" or a slightly different color, or grayer...but hair does come back.

What I (and my loved one) have learned was that Radiation treatments of the head, frequently kills the hair follicles on the scalp. Consequently this hair does not regenerate. It frequently will not come back after treatments. This hair loss is permanent.

[Again, I do NOT think the decision to proceed with Radiation should depend upon the risk of permanent hair loss, but it would give the Patient a more complete choice if she were informed *before* **treatment begins**, and maybe given a chance to plan ahead and think of her options for quality of life after treatment.]

The internet literature on hair loss is overwhelmingly about hair "thinning" due to age, demographics and genetics. It is difficult to find sources that address the issue of Medical Loss of Hair as a side effect of the toxicity of chemotherapy. I found it strange that so little information is available and so little was provided during our medical oncology experiences. It seems the two most talked about natural remedies are Provillus and Procerin; and of course, there are surgical alternatives.

[Visit: naturalhairlosstreatment.com,, provillus.com, .breastcancer.org, caring4cancer.com, .chemocare.com, and especially: www.tlcdirect.org the "Tender Loving Care" site of the American Cancer Society.]

Modesty:

Even as the Patient's cancer progresses, care should be taken by the Caregiver to be sensitive and respect the precious individuality of the Patient. For example, even if the Patient does not ask, the Caregiver should leave the bathroom area while the Patient engages in personal habits of hygiene or defecation just as they might have done so throughout the Patient's life. Peoples' modesty needs do not change. Give the Patient the space he/she is used to, for as long as you can. It is a clear signal of love and respect that will be appreciated.

Intimacy

All aspects of the Patient ⟷ Caregiver relationship are affected by the disease: intimacy and sexuality included. Of course, it is important to be sensitive to your Loved One's needs for attention and affection, and this sensitivity should extend to what is really appropriate given your Loved One's condition.

Imagine someone home from chemotherapy, who might be suffering from headaches, nausea, or stomach pain and diarrhea. The last thing imaginable to this person would be insensitive and inappropriate contact.
Cancer pushes couples to replace sexuality with affection. **It's all about her!**

It is important to FIND NEW WAYS to express intimacy—***a constant smile and sincere greeting like "Hello Beautiful,"*** sincere expressions of love (flowers, favorite sayings,...), light hugs, holding hands, or massaging your loved one's neck or achy muscles, reading a favorite book, or sharing a TV documentary, reading a spiritual book....basically giving your loved one the gifts of your ATTENTION, your TOUCH, your personal BEING.

As always, a kiss is still a kiss, and occasional flowers say it all. The essence of intimacy now must become *very fundamental: GIVING THE PATIENT A SENSE OF YOUR PRESENCE, YOUR AFFECTION, YOUR CONSTANCY, and YOUR SUPPORT.*

Caregiving during advanced stages of cancer is truly and authentically **SELF** – GIVING.

23)   Home Care Pitfalls / Safety:

Guidelines:
- Clear pathways for wheel chair/walker access,, unload firearms, remove throw rugs; remove bathroom rug when coming in with wheel chair;
- Falls Prevention; adequate lighting, night lights, shower chair, grab bars, run extension cords along wall or out from under foot, or cover extension cords; be vigilant using bedside commode;
- Fire safety: no smoking in bed, no open flames near Oxygen tanks, keep extinguisher handy;
- Environment: monitor weather reports, keep flashlights in working order, have extra food/water supplies;
- Medications: store meds out of reach of children, keep medications in original containers, take meds as instructed, follow med labels for correct dosages, record meds taken to avoid risk of overmedicating; never take someone else's medications.

[Source: Pathways Hospice, *Guide to Care*, p.12]

If professional Home Care is needed, the Caregiver should research to find the right Visiting Nurse or Home Care organization to fulfill this need; ask for neighbor experiences, check referrals, check your insurance to see what is covered.

Remember, in Home Care, ***strangers*** are coming into and sharing your personal spaces in your home.

You should meet and interview the people you let in. Check their ID badge. You will need to feel COMFORTABLE with each of them. If you feel uncomfortable, make up an excuse and ask them to leave.

Don't leave medications or valuables lying around out in the open. Caregivers and Patients should confer together, to discuss and <u>set **goals** to be achieved by professional Home Care</u>, and assess the value of the information and assistance received

24) <u>**Controls for Infection:**</u>

Medications and Chemotherapy may affect the marrow of your loved one's bones leading to low blood counts especially of the white blood cells

When your Partner's IMMUNE SYSTEM is weak, she will be very susceptible to INFECTIONS. As your Caregiver role requires a high priority on knowing and **managing side effects**, *equally as important are the* **controls for infection***.*

<u>**Hand Washing**</u>:   Most important of the controls for infection.

Wash your hands with soap and water *after* going to the bathroom, handling soiled linens or pajamas, handling garbage or food waste, or petting your pet dog or cat.

Wash your hands *before* you prepare medications, or prepare meals for your loved one.

A convenient alternative to soap and water is the alcohol "dry" hand purification techniques like Purell hand sanitizer, or wipes. I would recommend purchase of a few bottles, and strategically lay them around the house in locations where they are prominent and visible.

Frequent hand washing may leave them chapped and dry. Plan to have moisturizing lotions handy and use them often.

Decision Rule: When in doubt, wash your hands anyway.   I found it useful to overcome any sense of inconvenience of frequent hand washing, by dedicating the washing to her: "This one's for you."

<u>**Handling blood or bodily secretions:**</u>

Your Caregiver role may require you to handle blood, wound dressings, vomit, urine, stool, soiled linen or clothing---<u>Tough love</u>.

If you have latex gloves, wear them.   If you do not have latex gloves, wash the areas with clean paper towels and soapy water. Rinse. Place gloves and/or paper towels in a plastic bag and throw out into your home garbage can.

If any assistive devices are used, bedpans, commodes, vomit containers, wear gloves and flush contents down the toilet. Wash in hot soap and water in the tub or vanity, rinse. and dry with a disposable paper towel. Then **always wash your hands thoroughly after clean up**.

Dealing with Incontinence:

Incontinence—the inability to control the body's release of urine or stool—is another Tough Love matter. Incontinence may be due to age, or the cancer, or it may signal some pressure on the nerves from the tumor.

Incontinence is another embarrassing condition, much like diarrhea, making your loved one reticent to go out to social events, or visit friends or even family. We found a solution in the adult diapers, sold at all supermarkets. Called "briefs" these diapers usually are attached with Velcro strips, and easy to get on or off.
Have a large plastic bag handy, or plastic insert in your bathroom trash bag that has ties and can be sealed. Dispose of soiled briefs quickly to avoid noxious odors in the bathroom.

BE PATIENT with your loved one. This is something *beyond her control.* Be supportive. She felt more embarrassed and reticent than I did. I would reassure her that this was what was meant by "Better, or Worse" and would thank her for the opportunity to show her my constancy and affection.

Again, the body's natural immune system is very important in fighting infection. Especially important is the Patient's white blood cell count, since white blood cells role is fighting infection. Monitor the white blood count [WBC] in any blood draws. If your Patient is involved in strong chemotherapy, one side effect may be the lowering of white blood cells, putting your loved one **at high risk for infection**. You may want to ask your Oncologist if they have considered adding Neulasta into your loved one's chemo regimen; this drug is injected **1 day after** chemo treatment and stimulates white blood cell production.

---

25) CAREGIVER RELIEF FROM 24/7 COVERAGE:

A Flight Attendant stands in the front of the plane, and motions to the Exit locations, the instructions in the different warning lights, and finally, "If we experience a loss in cabin pressure, an Oxygen mask will drop out of the overhead console. <u>Put on **YOUR OWN** OXYGEN MASK FIRST, then install the second mask on your child</u>."

Caregiving for someone who is very ill is extremely intense and exhausting work. It can consume the Caregiver's attention and energy. It is brutally demanding. But, the bottom line is consistency. Your loved one needs and wants *to count on you to be there for her*, in all aspects of her life at this time. <u>Only you can give her all the holistic perspectives to her care—clinical, intellectual, emotional, spiritual.</u> Only you are there 24/7. You are her ROCK....and her compass.

And the really scary thing would be *you* cannot get ill, you cannot lose your purpose, you cannot undo the battle, you cannot turn your back. What would she do? Where would she go for help? You have to be "there for her" and your Presence is perhaps her sole comfort during these difficult times. You are the one who brings her comfort, hope, peace, acceptance, and even joy.

<u>You must take care of yourself, so you will be able to take care of your loved one</u>. It's as simple as that. <u>You cannot go down.</u>

> "Some days I am stressed beyond belief. Then other days I feel
> thankful for the time I have spent with my wife all these years.
> Then the next day, I feel angry that I have to juggle so much,
> and then I feel guilty for feeling angry. Basically, I never know
> how I'm going to feel one day to the next." ----Jim

> [cited in NCI, *When Someone you love has Advanced Cancer*, p.33]

And so it comes down to this; <u>you must be honest with yourself</u>. You need some breaks, some refreshing, some renewal, so you can come back to your loved one with new energy, new purpose, renewed strength, new laughter and joy to share and make her day a little brighter.

When *your loved one feels great frustration* with her condition, feels betrayed by her body, hates her constant fatigue, hates feeling sick, **she may lash out against you.** And why not? You are her rock. Who else can she lash out against? To whom else can she admit her depression, her "tired of being tired," her constant pain?

BE HER ROCK. Let it wash off your back. This is *frustration...*blowing off steam. It is not personal. *Let it go*.

I recall an incident where my loved one "dumped" on me, from frustration from her inability to move about on her own; it was her only mild rampage. I remember saying something like "Wow—that was a good one." **We both burst into laughter.** And it brought us so much closer together. And the cancer was beaten back for a couple of moments.

Caring for yourself means you get the strength to carry on. Taking time to recharge your own mind, body, and spirit helps *you* be a better Caregiver. Take time to break the intensity.

Some strategies for RELIEF and RENEWAL:
- connect with others, join a support group, connect with friends...
- let yourself laugh; find joy in hobbies or athletic endeavors....
- find some way to exercise your sense of play.....
- take a walk in the park, or around the block......
- read a book on the porch......
- write a journal, or collect pictures for a Life History Album......
- let go of mistakes, or guilt.........
- find some respite help so you can run errands....do chores.....
- take up photography...share your new pictures with your loved one......
- cook or barbeque a meal... share with friends....
- make something in the garage....change your car's oil....
- take up knitting, or sewing....make a scarf....
- bake a pie.......
- go to a movie..........
- read something spiritual or inspiring.......
- GO SHOPPING.......
- Make Time for Me........

If you can *FIND SOMETHING YOU ENJOY,* think of Nike's advertising slogan---
"*Just Do It*." and then *bring the joy back to your loved one*. Share your joy, and she will feel uplifted, and perhaps distracted for just a moment from the tedium of her battle with her cancer.

JOY begets JOY!

The Psychic Footprint of Cancer

In my contact with cancer patients and their families, the words they most commonly use to describe the experience are usually ... "devastated," "numb," "We never planned...."

This addresses the Greek notion of cancer as an *onkos* or *psychological burden*. Cancer can become obsessive. It gives the patient no escape. Relentless, it takes over thinking, enjoyment, excitement, enthusiasm. It can easily grow to become a dominating focus of the patient's life, and consequently, of the Caregiver's life as well.

Personal case:
In calendar 2009 **we experienced 116 separately billed medical interventions:** Office visits, clinic visits, one ER, one hospitalization, one four-month chemo = 81; Lab draws/analyses = 28; Imaging MRI, CT, mammography = 7 interventions. Side effects like baldness, weight loss, prosthetics—cancer seen daily in the mirror.

Cancer can get "in your face." Life can easily become a continuous focus on the next scheduled obligation. In this way cancer comes to steal living.......even years before it tries to steal *life*.

This is perhaps the Caregiver's most daunting challenge—to reframe what living is about, to reignite the spirit, to bring back splashes of joy, to inflame something of the zest for living, to find gratitude for the gifts living brings us on a daily basis---in a word, to RE-ENGAGE your loved one in LIFE, and find expressions of HOPE, and experiences of the JOY of LIVING each day---one day at a time.

I firmly believe you best fight the psychological burdens of cancer with LAUGHTER. That is why the concluding chapter of this book is on LAUGHTER.

This truly tests the *creativity* and *stamina* of the Caregiver.

Support Groups:

Your medical entity, Hospital or clinic, may have developed **Support Groups** where people undergoing the new experiences of cancer can meet, learn, and share information with others who are going through or who have completed the same experiences.

Most Cancer Centers have Caregiver Support Groups, Cancer Survivor Support Groups, a Prostate Cancer Support Group, and a Breast Cancer Support Group. Support Groups meet regularly and participate in educational seminars apropos to their group. If it is imperative to "learn as much as you can" this is a vehicle to achieve that goal, as well as provide emotional support for the members.

Support groups form their own bonds of friendship--your people, sharing your experience, sharing your journey. People you can call; people who can give you a needed ride; people sharing their adaptations to their cancer. Support Groups are a terrific source of information and solace. They walk the walk—with you.

Caregiver's Bill of Rights

I have the right to take care of myself. This is not an act of selfishness. It will give me the ability to take better care of my loved one.

I have the right to **seek help from others** even though my loved one may object. I know the limits of my own endurance and strength.

I have the right to **maintain parts of my own life** that do not include the person I care for, just as I would if she were healthy. I know that I do everything that I reasonably can for my loved one. I have the right to do some things just for myself.

I have the right to get angry, be depressed, and **express difficult feelings** once in a while.

I have the right to **reject any attempt** by my loved one to make me do things out of guilt or anger. It does not matter if she knows that she is doing it or not.

I have the right to get **consideration, affection, forgiveness, and acceptance** for what I do for my loved one, as I offer these in return.

I have the right to **take pride in what I am doing**. And I have the right to applaud the courage it has taken to meet the needs of my loved one.

I have the right to **protect my individuality**. I also have the right to a life that will sustain me in times when my loved one no longer needs my full-time help.

(Author Unknown)

[Source: National Cancer Institute, *When Someone You Love has Advanced Cancer*, p. 47]

26) <u>WHEN TO CALL FOR HELP:</u>

People usually fall into the Caregiver role, not by choice, but by circumstance. As the Patient's disease progresses, the demands on the Caregiver become more frequent and more intense. They tend to creep up unnoticed until they are so excessive they harm the Caregiver's ability to assist his loved one.

In an article on "Being a Caregiver"

"Caregivers often lose themselves in giving good care. As a Caregiver, you may be so focused on the Patient that you forget about your own needs. Little by little you may have given up activities and outside interests, and even your own health may be affected. In order to take care of your loved one, it's essential for you to take care of yourself. Basic self-care includes finding time to rest, eating well, and getting some exercise."

Suggestions for Caregivers
- **Get enough rest.** If you don't sleep well at night, take a nap when your loved one is resting.
- **Exercise** is a stress reliever. A short walk can do wonders for your wellbeing.
- **Take breaks** whenever possible. Go for coffee with a friend. Even a short break can help.
- **Set priorities and take one thing at a time**. Divide tasks into manageable parts.
- **Keep lists** that help you track what needs to be done and also help you delegate tasks.
- **Talk** about your concerns and feelings with a trusted friend or a member of the [medical] team.
- **Ask for help** from other family members or friends, as well as the [medical] team."

[Source: Pathways Hospice, *Dying Is...* p.19]

The Caregiver should prepare for the eventuality that care must now be provided in a medical environment, with competent medical personnel available 24/7, and with medical technology and equipment readily available.

This realization came for me when my loved one could no longer stand upright *on her own*. and became a *dead weight*, I could not hold her upright and still reach down and pull up her pajama bottoms. I knew then that <u>I needed additional help</u> to be able to provide adequate care for her. I could no longer do this by myself.

Call for "Help" ***before*** situations get out of hand. Talk these issues over with the Oncology Team. A Caregiver can benefit from their experience to guide these types of decisions.

----

27) **FINAL NOTE: Thoughts on LAUGHTER**

"Good morning Beautiful."

Every day, every morning, I would greet her with a *smile* and *this phrase*. And she would *smile* in return. She told me she *looked forward to each morning*--kicked off with our exchange of smiles. And the real marvel of it was we both knew the other meant it. This would begin each day with this note of joy...that set the tone for the remainder of our *adventures* together—on that new day, one-day-at-a-time. Everything would cascade from this greeting.

We had been doing this for years—even after the diagnosis of *metastatic cancer* throughout her spinal column, pelvis, moving upward to become brain lesions, the mastectomy, and the baldness due to whole head radiation, the emaciated physique. *All the major physical characteristics that make a woman feel beautiful---gone.* What extraordinary courage—to find *joy* in spite of her condition. She looked more beautiful now than when we were married.

My loved one began a journal back in 2006 when we found out her cancer had spread to her bones. She called it her "*Joy Journal.*" She decided to record instances of *joy* even in the face of advanced cancer, so she could look back on them later, and re-experience some of the brighter moments of her life with a brutal, terminal disease. *These fleeting moments of joy became sacred, spiritual moments for both of us.*

The first few lines that began her *Joy Journal* were:

> *"Someday, I will design a quilt of my life.....whimsical, musical, and*
> *magical.....the colors calming to the soul; the patterns bringing smiles*
> *to the children I have touched....*
> *This journal is dedicated to the Joy life brings me each day."*

And the final entry:

> *"I have found the magic of following my heart..... I cherish my life."*

An Excerpt from her Journal:

"July 30, 2009" Most joyful event "Walking with Dinosaurs" We went over to the Pepsi Center for the outstanding presentation. It was so exciting I felt like a kid at my first puppet show. The sweetest part was I kept saying I wanted to go with no response from John, Then he surprised me with tickets. Joy-Joy-Joy-Joy."

I have learned that **JOY emanates from the depths of one's being.** And **developing a sense of humor** may be one of the most important lessons a human being can learn in this life.

The outward expression of JOY is LAUGHTER, and laughter has tremendous healing properties. When laughter is shared it binds people together and increases intimacy. Humor and laughter are powerful antidotes to pain, stress, and conflict. Laughter strengthens the body's immune system, boosts energy, diminishes pain, and protects the body from the harmful and damaging effects of stress. Laughter truly is good medicine!

A very recent study at the University of Maryland Medical Center in Baltimore shows that Laughter and a Sense of Humor provide serious protection of the vascular system, and prevent heart attacks. In this study laughter caused the vascular endothelial tissues to dilate 22% bringing more blood cells and oxygen to the various tissues of the body; conversely, stress caused a 35% constriction of the endothelium. The head cardiologist and researcher, Dr. Michael Miller is quoted in the article as saying "The (medical) recommendations for heart health may one day be: *exercise*, *eat right*, *and laugh* a few times a day."

[See: University of Maryland Medical Center,
www.umm.edu/features/laughter.htm]

Benefits of Laughter:

Physical Benefits	Mental Health Benefits	Social Benefits
boosts immunity	expresses joy, zest for life	strengthens relationships
lowers stress hormones	eases anxiety and fear	attracts others
decreases pain	relieves stress	enhances teamwork
relaxes muscles	improves mood	helps defuse conflict
prevents heart attack	enhances resilience	promotes bonding

- Laughter relaxes the whole body. relieving physical tension and stress, leaving the muscles relaxed.
- Laughter boosts the immune system, by decreasing stress hormones and increasing immune cells.
- Laughter releases endorphins, the body's natural "feel good" chemicals; endorphins promote the sense of well-being, and trigger the pituitary gland to release its own opiates which temporarily relieve pain.
- Laughter protects the heart and vascular health, by improving the function of the blood vessels, increasing blood flow and oxygenation of tissues.

William Fry MD, of Stanford University describes how **humor** and its consequent *laughter* involve the entire brain, since their intellectual source is incongruity—creating a relationship between disconnected items.

> "Humor works quickly. Less than a half-second after exposure to something funny (like a joke), electrical waves move through the higher brain functions of the cerebral cortex. The left hemisphere analyzes the words and structures of the joke; the right hemisphere "gets" the joke; the visual sensory area of the occipital lobe creates images; the limbic (emotional) system makes you happier; and the motor sections (of your brain) make you smile or laugh."

> [Visit www.helpguide.org/life/humor_laughter-health.htm and www.care2.com//]

I have learned that **joy**---and its expression **in laughter** or at least **a smile**---can be the most important guardian of a loving relationship.

I was in the Waiting Lounge at the Cancer Rehab Institute where I overheard a conversation between two student physical therapists who were talking about a boy one of them had met the weekend before. They did not seem to care that anyone in the room could not help but overhear their conversation. One asked the other student how does one tell if this could be the beginning of a real relationship?

When the second student left, I could not contain myself.
I asked her "Does he make you laugh?"

She was caught off guard, and stammered.
I told her life brings the unexpected, and if either one of them were ever debilitated by some condition like the cancer that brought us to the Rehab Institute, it will be their capacity to find ***splashes of joy and laughter***--- ***even then***. That is what gives a relationship its ***strength to carry through.***

Don't worry about love; make *laughter* the indicator for a successful future relationship.

I have learned that a **_smile_** is the "feel good" **_predisposition_** to laughter. Just flashing a smile tells everyone around you that you are o.k., that you acknowledge them and hope they are o.k. as well.

A smile is a **_self-fulfilling_** energy; it is the stepping stone to a deeper experience of joy or laughter. It disposes you to be in a receptive attitude, to be friendly and concerned about the other. It propels you forward into feeling good about yourself and others. It signals that you wish someone else well. A smile tells the world, and your loved one, that you are glad to see her. There is a promise of magic behind a smile.
Remember the cliche' "A smile is language that even a baby understands." Universally true.

I have learned that joy begets a sense of **_playfulness_**. Playing together is sharing the joy each brings to the game. Playing brings people together; playing strengthens the bond between the partners and even their opponents. And the focus becomes enjoying each other and the game itself. Wasn't there a Great Teacher who said, "Unless you become as little children...."?
We are never too old to play together. The joy in play keeps one thinking young.
My challenge was to keep trying to build in playfulness, and enjoyment into her life, any way that I could creatively do so Playfulness distracts your loved one, and pushes away her cancer for a moment. Playfulness spawns laughter.

In Conlusion

I have learned that the GREATEST GIFTS my loved one and I gave to each other come down to living in the moment while seeing life as an _adventure_, not taking ourselves or the world too seriously, and _laughing together_ along the way.

We created the kind of life that she called "......_whimsical, musical,.....magical_."

We loved and lived the magic in our lives. **_We found joy in nearly everything we did._**

Nothing seemed impossible to us.

Nothing could stop us----except cancer.

EXHIBITS

CANCER PATIENT NAME   **Subject: MEDICATIONS LIST:**

Cancer Overview:

[1] Daily Medications:

       History ....

[2] Chemotherapy: differing Weekly Intervals ~ Infusion therapy and injections—

       History: --

[3] As needed:

ONCOLOGIST: _Dr._ _____ _Phone_ _____

                                  _____ _Updated02/10/2010_

CANCER PATIENT NAME   Subject: **MEDICATIONS LIST**

Overview: Breast Cancer diagnosed: 2/01, [lumpectomy, AC chemo. No radia.] ; Metastasis: 2/06 [r. mastectomy, metal pins l. femur, r. humerus,] chemo; 6/08 [brain radia+chemo]; 10/09 chemo; 1/15/10 brain radiation per MRI.

[1] *Daily:*   *Vitamins Supplement* -- *Women's One-a-Day*
                        Calcium -- (750mg supplement + D)
                        B-Complex -- (stimulate immune system/manage stress)
                        Prednisone (5mg) –(for Scleroderma joint inflammation)
                        Protonix (40 mg) -- (esophagus/upper GI discomfort)
                        Citalopram HBR (20mg) – (for depression) ~ 2/12/10

    History ....

      Lapatinib (Tykerb) [1250mg (5 tablets)] -- (protein-tyrosine kinase estrogen recep. inhibitor) ~
                            (begun 10/08)
                        Letrozole (Femara)   aromatase inhibitor (2002-2006 and 6/09; discontinued: 9/9/09 pending new
                            regimen of chemotherapy)
                        Aromasin (Exemestane) (25 mg) estrogen receptor inhibitor(begun 10/2007)   (disctd 06/04/08)
                        Megestrol (Megace) [160 mg (4 tablets) ~estrogen recp inhibitor (begun 01/09, disctd 05/31/09)

[2] ***Chemotherapy: differing Weekly Intervals ~ Infusion therapy*** and ***injections*—**
                        Zometa -- (bone restoration) ~ (begun: 05/05/06) [every 3rd wk)
                        Neulasta (injection) ~ as needed for low WBC production

    History ....
                        Ixabepilone (Ixempra) IV ~ begun: 09/16/09; disc 1/20/10 [3wks]
                        Fulvestrant (Faslodex) – estrogen receptor antagonist for metastic
                            breast cancer (begun: 07/03/06; discontinued 05/14/08).
                        Herceptin (Trastuzumab)   ~ HER-2 estrogen receptor inhibitor (begun: 07/03/06)
                            (discontinued 06/04/08).
                        Paclitaxel (Abraxane) - (begun 07/07/08; dosage modified
                            from 460mg/3 wks to 300mg/2wks) (discontinued: 10/6/08)

[3] *As needed*:   Ativan -- (for specific stress situations)
                        Compazine (10 mg) -- (nausea related to radiation)
                        MiraLax -- (for constipation)
                        Immodium -- (for diarrhea as needed)

ONCOLOGIST   *Dr. xxxxx xxxxxx, Med Oncologist,   xxxxxx Cancer Center*
                        ~ Telephone: xxx-xxx-xxxx

                                   Updated 02/10/2010

CANCER PATIENT   Lab Results

Date of Draw:	WBC	RBC	Hgb	AST	Marker CEA	Weight

| CANCER PATIENT | | | | | Lab Results @ McKee | |

Date:	WBC	RBC	Hgb	AST	CEA	Weight
7/3/2008	3.8	3.73	11.5	111	334	147
7/16/2008	10.1	3.69	11.5		20.4	
8/8/2008				29		
8/22/2008	11.7	3.54	11.3	35		144
9/4/2008	17.4	3.36	10.8	33	5.1	139
9/18/2008	13.4	2.97	10	28	2.9	142
10/2/2008	12	2.64	9	28	1.3	
10/31/2008				36	1.7	143
11/26/2008	4.6	3.81	12.1		4.3	
12/24/2008	5.9	3.77	11.7	38	13.1	142
1/20/2009	5.7	3.66	11.7	35	35.1	139
2/19/2009	7.1	3.7	11.8	38	48.2	
3/19/2009	8.5	3.85	12.5	54	62.3	137
4/16/2009	6	3.62	11.8	44	74.4	
5/15/2009	5.6	3.42	11.3	56	93.5	
7/10/2009	5.8	3.42	11.1	78	119	135
8/7/2009	5.1	3.36	10.7	118		
8/31/2009	5.6	3.54	11	165	203	137
10/16/2009	8.8	3.6	11.2	68	182	133
10/28/2009	6.9	3.38	10.5	51	113	
11/18/2009	5.8	3.39	10.6	36	46.2	
12/9/2009	6.4	3.48	11.1	43	23.7	129
12/29/2009	6.4	3.4	10.9	35	21.9	130
1/15/2010	6.8	3.46	11.1	52	25.4	124

Interpretation: Note the following: Column 1: note the low white blood counts (WBC), which indicate my partner was chronically susceptible to infection [Caregiver Warning Flag].

By following the marker numbers in Column 6, the reader can see that we began (7/3/08) with a very high CEA. We began chemotherapy and knocked it down to the "normal" range of <5 for a few months (09 thru 12). But the cancer came back throughout her body, and we decided to begin a fifth round of chemo in September, 09. We knocked the cancer back, but could not obtain a marker range below 22. Our Oncologist decided to obtain an MRI to find out why.

The MRI revealed several large lesions in the brain, one impacting the cerebellum and the brain stem. Inoperable. The Oncology Team suggested brain radiation to try to shrink this large tumor. and then try pinpoint (stereotactic) radiation to try to kill the tumor. The tumor did not respond and within a month became the proximate cause of her demise.
These numbers tell the Clinical side of her story.

Exhibit 3

Meds Log

DATE	8-9am	10-11am	12-1pm	2-3pm	4-5pm	6-7pm	8-9pm	10-11pm	Comment
	Meds	Meds	Meds	Meds	Meds	Meds	Meds	Meds	

Caregiver Internet Sources

Rating	Internet Site	Comments
5 *****	WebMD.com	Starting point for all personal medical research...user friendly site.
5 *****	MedicineNet.com	Excellent on all types of meds. Cross-references WebMD.
4 ****	Am Cancer Society <cancer.org>	Best overall compendium of information, resources, esp."Caregivers" key link to TLC <tlcdirect.org>
4 ****	National Cancer Institute <cancer.gov>	Good on resrach, clinical trials, pipeline meds, treatments. etc.
4 ****	Medifocus.com	Guidebooks on the major serious medical conditions...cancers...etc
4 ****	Breast Cancer.org	Great on new and targeted therapies...new meds coming on line...
4 ****	Coping w/ Cancer <copingmag.com>	Excellent articles for Caregivers--good articles on Side Effects.
4 ****	aan.com (Am Acad of Neurology)	Excellent site on Caregiving for Neurological diseases, incl cancer
3 ***	RxList.com	Good for specific meds, (tied to WebMD.) Excellent med reviews
3 ***	Founda for Health Care Coverage (CA) <coverageforall.org>	Interesting site on insurance, and resources, localized by State MATRIX
3 ***	Caring4Cancer.com	Pretty good on clinical trials...new stuff
3 ***	Amer Assoc for Cancer Research <aacrjournals.org>	Clinical research...starting to get too technical for layman.... includes Clinical Cancer Research
3 ***	Amer Brain Tumor Assoc <abta.org>	Excellent on Brain Tumor specific info, good Caregiver study... [05/2010]
2 **	Journal of Clinical Oncology <ascopubs.org>	Over my head, but one can ascertain the "gist" of the article and get an idea of what is being looked at by cancer researchers...
2 **	ChemoCare.com	Interesting anecdotes....
2 **	coverColorado.org	Insurance for people with pre-existing conditions.

Exhibit 5

2010 POVERTY GUIDELINES*
ALL STATES (EXCEPT ALASKA AND HAWAII) AND D.C.

ANNUAL GUIDELINES

FAMILY SIZE	PERCENT OF POVERTY GUIDELINE								
	100%	120%	133%	135%	150%	175%	185%	200%	250%
1	10,830.00	12,996.00	14,403.90	14,620.50	16,245.00	18,952.50	20,035.50	21,660.00	27,075.00
2	14,570.00	17,484.00	19,378.10	19,669.50	21,855.00	25,497.50	26,954.50	29,140.00	36,425.00
3	18,310.00	21,972.00	24,352.30	24,718.50	27,465.00	32,042.50	33,873.50	36,620.00	45,775.00
4	22,050.00	26,460.00	29,326.50	29,767.50	33,075.00	38,587.50	40,792.50	44,100.00	55,125.00
5	25,790.00	30,948.00	34,300.70	34,816.50	38,685.00	45,132.50	47,711.50	51,580.00	64,475.00
6	29,530.00	35,436.00	39,274.90	39,865.50	44,295.00	51,677.50	54,630.50	59,060.00	73,825.00
7	33,270.00	39,924.00	44,249.10	44,914.50	49,905.00	58,222.50	61,549.50	66,540.00	83,175.00
8	37,010.00	44,412.00	49,223.30	49,963.50	55,515.00	64,767.50	68,468.50	74,020.00	92,525.00

For family units of more than 8 members, add $3,740 for each additional member.

MONTHLY GUIDELINES

FAMILY SIZE	PERCENT OF POVERTY GUIDELINE								
	100%	120%	133%	135%	150%	175%	185%	200%	250%
1	902.50	1,083.00	1,200.33	1,218.38	1,353.75	1,579.38	1,669.63	1,805.00	2,256.25
2	1,214.17	1,457.00	1,614.84	1,639.13	1,821.25	2,124.79	2,246.21	2,428.33	3,035.42
3	1,525.83	1,831.00	2,029.36	2,059.88	2,288.75	2,670.21	2,822.79	3,051.67	3,814.58
4	1,837.50	2,205.00	2,443.88	2,480.63	2,756.25	3,215.63	3,399.38	3,675.00	4,593.75
5	2,149.17	2,579.00	2,858.39	2,901.38	3,223.75	3,761.04	3,975.96	4,298.33	5,372.92
6	2,460.83	2,953.00	3,272.91	3,322.13	3,691.25	4,306.46	4,552.54	4,921.67	6,152.08
7	2,772.50	3,327.00	3,687.43	3,742.88	4,158.75	4,851.88	5,129.13	5,545.00	6,931.25
8	3,084.17	3,701.00	4,101.94	4,163.63	4,626.25	5,397.29	5,705.71	6,168.33	7,710.42

Produced by: CMSO/DEHPG/DEEO

In accordance with section 1012 of the Department of Defense Appropriations Act of 2010, the poverty guidelines published on January 23, 2009 willl remain in effect until updated poverty guidelines are published in March 2010.

Exhibit 6

ADVANCE DIRECTIVE FOR MEDICAL / SURGICAL TREATMENT
(Living Will)

On completion, give copies to your physician, family members, and Healthcare Agent. If you wish to revoke or replace this document, mark it clearly as "Revoked" or destroy it and all its copies, if possible. If you do not understand the choices and options, seek advice from a healthcare provider or other qualified advisor.

I. DECLARATION

I, _____, am at least eighteen years old and able to make and communicate my own decisions. It is my direction that the following instructions be followed if I am diagnosed by two qualified doctors to be in a terminal condition or Persistent Vegetative State.

A. Terminal Condition

If at any time my physician and one other qualified physician certify in writing that I have a terminal condition, and I am unable to make or communicate my own decisions about medical treatment, then:

1. Life-Sustaining Procedures *(initial one)*:

_____ *(Initials)* I direct that all life-sustaining procedures shall be withdrawn and/or withheld, not including any procedure considered necessary by my healthcare providers to provide comfort or relieve pain.

_____ *(Initials)* I direct that life-sustaining procedures shall be continued for/until *(state timeframe or goal)*:

_____

2. Artificial Nutrition and Hydration

If I am receiving nutrition and hydration by tube, I direct that one of the following actions be taken *(initial one)*:

_____ *(Initials)* Artificial nutrition and hydration shall not be continued.

_____ *(Initials)* Artificial nutrition and hydration shall be continued for/until *(state timeframe or goal)*:

_____

_____ *(Initials)* Artificial nutrition and hydration shall be continued, if medically possible and advisable according to my healthcare providers.

B. Persistent Vegetative State

If at any time my physician and one other qualified physician certify in writing that I am in a Persistent Vegetative State, then:

1. Life-Sustaining Procedures *(initial one)*:

_____ *(Initials)* I direct that life-sustaining procedures shall be withdrawn and/or withheld, not including any procedure considered necessary by my healthcare providers to provide comfort or relieve pain.

_____ *(Initials)* I direct that life-sustaining procedures shall be continued for/until *(state timeframe or goal)*:

_____

2. Artificial Nutrition and Hydration

If I am receiving nutrition and hydration by tube, I direct that one of the following actions be taken *(initial one)*:

_____ *(Initials)* Artificial nutrition and hydration shall not be continued.

_____ *(Initials)* Artificial nutrition and hydration shall be continued for/until *(state timeframe or goal)*:

_____

_____ *(Initials)* Artificial nutrition and hydration shall be continued, if medically possible and advisable according to my healthcare providers.

II. OTHER DIRECTIONS

Please indicate below if you have attached to this form any other instructions for your care after you are certified in a terminal condition or Persistent Vegetative State *(for instance, to be enrolled in a hospice program, remain at or be transferred to home, discontinue or refuse other treatments such as dialysis, transfusions, antibiotics, diagnostic tests, etc.) (initial one)*:

_____ *(Initials)* Yes, I have attached other directions.

_____ *(Initials)* No, I do not have any other directions.

III. RESOLUTION WITH MEDICAL POWER OF ATTORNEY *(initial one)*

_____ *(Initials)* My Agent under my Medical Durable Power of Attorney shall have the authority to override any of the directions stated here, whether I signed this declaration before or after I appointed that Agent.

_____ *(Initials)* My directions as stated here may not be overridden or revoked by my Agent under Medical Durable Power of Attorney, whether I signed this declaration before or after I appointed that Agent.

Exhibit 6

IV. CONSULTATION WITH OTHER PERSONS

I authorize my healthcare providers to discuss my condition and care with the following persons, understanding that these persons are not empowered to make any decisions regarding my care, unless I have appointed them as my Healthcare Agents under Medical Durable Power of Attorney.

Name   *Relationship*

_____

_____

_____

_____

V. NOTIFICATION OF OTHER PERSONS

Before withholding or withdrawal life-sustaining procedures, my healthcare providers shall make a reasonable effort to notify the following persons that I am in a terminal condition or Persistent Vegetative State. My healthcare providers have my permission to discuss my condition with these persons. I do NOT authorize these persons to make medical decisions on my behalf, unless I have appointed one or more of them as my Agent(s) under Medical Durable Power of Attorney.

Name   *Telephone number or email*

_____

_____

_____

VI. ANATOMICAL GIFTS

_____ (*Initials*) I wish to donate my (*check one or both*)
_____ organs and/or _____ tissues, if medically possible.

_____ (*Initials*) I do not wish donate my organs or tissues.

VII. SIGNATURE

I execute this declaration, as my free and voluntary act, this_____day of _____, 20____.

_____

Declarant signature

VIII. DECLARATION OF WITNESSES

This declaration was signed by (*name of Declarant*)

_____

in our presence, and we, in the presence of each other, and at the Declarant's request, have signed our names below as witnesses. We declare that, at the time the Declarant signed this declaration, we believe that he or she was of sound mind and under no pressure or undue influence. We did not sign the Declarant's signature. We are not doctors or employees of the attending doctor or healthcare facility in which the Declarant is a patient. We are neither creditors nor heirs of the Declarant and have no claim against any portion of the Declarant's estate at the time this declaration was signed. We are at least eighteen (18) years old and under no pressure, undue influence, or otherwise disqualifying disability.

_____

Signature of Witness

_____

Printed Name

_____

Address

_____

_____

Signature of Witness

_____

Printed Name

_____

Address

_____

Notary Seal (optional)

State of _____

County of _____ }

SUBSCRIBED and sworn to before me by

_____, the Declarant,

and _____

and _____

witnesses, as the voluntary act and deed of the Declarant

this day of _____, 20____.

_____

Notary Public
My commission expires:_____

Exhibit 7

MEDICAL DURABLE POWER OF ATTORNEY FOR HEALTHCARE DECISIONS

I. APPOINTMENT OF AGENT AND ALTERNATES

I, _____ ,
Declarant, hereby appoint:

_____
Name of Agent

_____
Agent's Best Contact Telephone Number

_____
Agent's email or alternative telephone number

_____
Agent's home address

as my Agent to make and communicate my healthcare decisions when I cannot. This gives my Agent the power to consent to, or refuse, or stop any healthcare, treatment, service, or diagnostic procedure. My Agent also has the authority to talk with healthcare personnel, get information, and sign forms as necessary to carry out those decisions.

If the person named above is not available or is unable to continue as my Agent, then I appoint the following person(s) to serve in the order listed below.

_____
Name of Alternate Agent #1

_____
Agent's Best Contact Telephone Number

_____
Agent's email or alternative telephone number

_____
Agent's home address

_____
Name of Alternate Agent #2

_____
Agent's Best Contact Telephone Number

_____
Agent's email or alternative telephone number

_____
Agent's home address

II. WHEN AGENT'S POWERS BEGIN

By this document, I intend to create a Medical Durable Power of Attorney which shall take effect either (*initial one*):

_____ (*Initials*) Immediately upon my signature.

_____ (*Initials*) When my physician or other qualified medical professional has determined that I am unable to make my or express my own decisions, and for as long as I am unable to make or express my own decisions.

III. INSTRUCTIONS TO AGENT

My Agent shall make healthcare decisions as I direct below, or as I make known to him or her in some other way. If I have not expressed a choice about the decision or healthcare in question, my Agent shall base his or her decisions on what he or she, in consultation with my healthcare providers, determines is in my best interest. I also request that my Agent, to the extent possible, consult me on the decisions and make every effort to enable my understanding and find out my preferences.

State here any desires concerning life-sustaining procedures, treatment, general care and services, including any special provisions or limitations:

_____
_____
_____
_____
_____
_____
_____
_____
_____
_____

My signature below indicates that I understand the purpose and effect of this document:

_____
Signature of Declarant   *Date*

Pursuant to Colorado Revised Statute 15-14.503–509   87   [www.coloradoadvancedirectives.com/MDPOA_form.pdf]

Exhibit 8

Medicare Health Plans in Colorado with *OUT OF POCKET LIMIT:*	Plan Type	Prescription Drugs Covered	Phone Number
AETNA Medicare (family coverage)			800-455-1560
Premiere	PPO	Yes	
Standard	PPO	Yes	
AETNA Medicare			800-455-1560
Premiere	HMO	Yes	
Value	HMO	Yes	
ANTHEM BlueCross/Blue Shield			800-797-1746
Sure Value Plus	HMO	Yes	
Smart Value Classic	PFFS	No	800-797-6419
Smart Value Plus	PFFS	Yes	800-797-6419
High Deductible (PERACare)	PPO	Yes	800-737-2258
CIGNA Medicare Access	PFFS	No	800-577-9409
(Plus Rx)	PFFS	Yes	
COLORADO Access	HMO	Yes	877-287-6767
HUMANA Gold Plus	HMO	33%	800-833-2364
Choice 005	PPO	Yes	
Choice 006 (Select counties)	PPO	No	
Gold Choice	PFFS	33%	
KAISER Permanente Senior Advan.			800-509-7570
Core	HMO	Yes	
Gold	HMO	Yes	
Plus Choice	HMO	Yes	
Silver	HMO	Yes	
ROCKY MOUNTAIN Health Plans			800-346-4643
Plus (Cost)	Cost	No	
Standard	Cost	No	
Green + Rx	Cost	Yes	
SECURE HORIZONS UnitedHealthcare			800-547-5514
AARP Med Complete Plans	HMO	Yes	
STERLING LIFE Insurance Co			888-858-8572
Basic Plus Segment 3	PFFS	No	
Option IV	PFFS	Yes	

Anthem ✚💠

EXPLANATION OF BENEFITS

ISSUE DATE	PAGE	E002868
February 1, 2010	00001 OF 00002	

Important for HSA

```
||||||||||||||||||||||||||||||||||||||
*******************AUT
22780 1 AT 0.357
████████
LOVELAND CO  80538-92i
```

> This is an EOB for imaging services received: MRI of the brain.
>
> This was BEFORE we had met our HDHP Deductible for the 2010 Plan year. So we are required to pay everything up to the Deductible first.; then 20% until we reach the Out-of-Pocket maximum.
>
> Notice that the Hospital billed our insurance $3,792.90; but because of contracted discounts, the amount to be paid is only $1,494.32. Always let your primary insurance work first; then you can calculate your liability, and note the primary actuallly does it for you. Liability: $1,494.32.

Patient's Name: ████████
Claim Number: 10027CD0511
Claim Processed Date: 02/01/10   Patient Acct. Number: ████████

Paid Amount: $0.00
It is your responsibility to pay: $1,494.32 It is not your responsibility to pay: $2,298.58
Thank you for using a Network Participating Provider

SERVICE DATE(s)	TYPE OF SERVICE	TOTAL BILLED	OTHER AMOUNT(S)	PATIENT SAVINGS	APPLIED TO DEDUCTIBLE	COINSURANCE COPAYMENT AMOUNT	CLAIMS PAYMENT
01/21/10	Drugs-Radiology	376.50		45.18/01	331.32/02		0.00
01/21/10	Magnetic Resonance	3,416.40		2,253.40/01	1,163.00/02		0.00
	TOTAL THIS CLAIM	3,792.90	0.00	2,298.58	1,494.32	0.00	0.00

Member's MEDICAL & PRESCRIPTION Deductible applied to date: $1,678.63

DETAIL MESSAGE:
01 – This is the amount in excess of the allowed expense for a participating provider. The member, therefore, is not responsible for this amount.
02 – This amount has been applied to the member's medical deductible.

HAVE QUESTIONS??
Check out our Website at WWW.ANTHEM.COM
Order I.D. Cards / Check claims status / Review benefits /
Verify family members covered on your policy / Find a participating provider
OR call our CUSTOMER SERVICE DEPARTMENT AT: 1-877-737-2258

MAIL ALL INQUIRIES   ANTHEM BLUE CROSS AND BLUE SHIELD
OR CLAIMS TO :   P.O. BOX 5747
                    DENVER, CO 80217-5747

WE SUGGEST THAT YOU RETAIN THIS COPY FOR YOUR INCOME TAX RECORDS.

THIS IS NOT A BILL

NUTRITION LOG

S M T W Th F S   Date: _____   *Comments*

7-9am [Bkfst]		

10-11am		

Noon [Lunch]		

2-3pm		

4-6pm [Dinner]		

7-9pm		

Weight _____

Observations:

NUTRITION LOG

S M (T) W Th F S   Date: **8/5** _____   **Comments**

Time	Food	
7-9am [Bkfst]	Soft boiled egg + 1 Toast + jelly	✓
10-11am	Water + pills	✓
Noon [Lunch]	—	
2-3pm	Banana milk shake + ½ Vanilla Inst. Breakfast	Ⓡ ↓
4-6pm [Dinner]	—	
7-9pm	water + pills	✓

Weight [   ]

Observations: Ⓡeaction

Combination of banana milkshake plus ½ Instant Breakfast was too rich for her system — lead to diarrhea.

91

EPILOGUE

END OF LIFE: Preparing for the Future

Your loved one may not yet be in this sunset stage of her life, but YOU should begin to think about whatever the future may bring, so you will be prepared for any eventuality.

Let's get the numbers out of the way.

According to a 2010 funeral price survey by the National Funeral Directors Association, the U.S. average cost for an adult funeral is $7,775.00, including casket and vault. Cemetery costs including grave stone marker may add $1000 and up. Therefore the average traditional funeral and burial will run roughly around $8,775.00.   Cremation runs from about $1,000.00 (simple) up to $10,000. (full service with memorial service and burial.)

This can be a serious hardship on the family, unless there has been some planning ahead. *Your loved one will certainly want to spare her family any financial burden.*

 You may feel it is too early in your loved one's diagnosis to even consider thinking about these things.   My recommendation is to begin to research options now, rather than put it off and *have to do it* when you are overwhelmed fighting grief and mental numbness at a later time. ***Do it now*** while your thinking is clear.   [Visit www.funeralwise.com, or Google search the topic]

Learn that costs can usually be negotiated, and many funeral homes will accept installment arrangements.

Your medical insurance will not cover funeral costs. You may want to research supplemental low benefit life insurance options (say $10,000) specifically for this purpose.

I know this is hard.   This is tough love. We are not culturally accustomed to address these issues. We "think young" in this country. These realities are uncomfortable to talk about.   But that is exactly why we—as a nation—are so *unprepared* for these eventualities. And the financial consequences can be devastating.   Be the Rock. Do this now. ***Get information.*** .

92

END OF LIFE : Hope changes to Acceptance Strategies:

There comes a time when your Patient realizes she has so much to overcome and is so weak or burnt out from years of fighting the disease, the realities of its progression and its finality begin to sink in. *Depression* is a natural progression in her mental state at this time. It reflects her growing realization of our universal human mortality.

A common phenomenon of this end stage of life is that _**both**_ the Caregiver and Patient _**know**_ _**they are approaching the end of life**_, but they are reluctant to talk about their feelings or their worries because <u>each does not want to cause the other sorrow or pain</u>. It is a tacit stand-off.

If you see a furled brow ask her if anything is worrying her. My best advice is to allow your loved one to bring up what she is worrying about. After all <u>it's all about her</u> at this point in time. Reassure her **you** will be o.k.   It gives her permission to leave.

Hope always looks into the FUTURE

Hope still holds out promise---for a possible cure, or some form of relief, or a "miracle."

When cure appears no longer probable, *focus shifts more to the short term*. We talk about "living in the moment.," and the cancer Patient with her Caregiver now look for new COPING STRATEGIES or skills that will allow the cancer Patient to "make do" and live on with her cancer.... survive with new obstacles to overcome. This is a natural progression of hope.

There will come a time when it becomes *patently clear that there will be no Patient cure, no Patient remission, no Patient recovery from the ravages of her cancer, no "miracle."*

This realization will slowly move the Caregiver *beyond denial*, and require the Caregiver to face the reality and finality of his loved one's limited life expectancy.

Caregiver and Patient may think thoughts like "we can make it with home care, or we will get a hospital bed, or maybe a nursing home."   And this lulls the Partners into a sense that they can "make it *somehow*".... albeit harder and harder to do so. We call this the "will to live" and "fighting" has been *your loved one's response to the disease throughout its duration*. It is ingrained into her nature. We say "she is a fighter."

Moving through this last ray of Hope *is not giving up or hopelessness*; it is a last-ditch mild form of denial. She will move through it to Acceptance, and so must her Caregiver. Be strong; ease and reinforce her movement to Acceptance.

It is now *totally about her*. <u>*Peace will be your last gift to your loved one.*</u>

Concentration by patient and caregiver on the *coping urgencies of the present moment* may tunnel their vision, and crowd hope (about the *future*) onto a back burner of consciousness. Any *new information, if* about a stabilization of your loved one's condition or a new coping strategy, can rekindle embers of hope and bring them out to a front burner of awareness. But over time, living in the moment takes over.

Hope now shifts to become Acceptance;. and ***Acceptance brings deep inner PEACE, and drives out FEAR.***

<u>Acceptance looks to the PRESENT MOMENT, and sees WHAT IS</u>. In Acceptance, the person sees what the present moment calls for, and embraces it. Acceptance means

> <u>***"For NOW, this is what this situation, this moment, requires me to do,
>   and so I do it willingly."***</u>
>
> [E. Tolle, *A New Earth*, p.296]

<u>Acceptance does not mean *giving up*</u>; it is not like resignation; <u>it is an</u> ***active choice***--- a choice to actively *embrace the present moment* with its present exigencies, with its inevitability, with its finality. *It is what it is.*

<u>This determination is made by your loved one at the deepest center of her Being, and it brings her deep inner PEACE.   It puts your loved one in touch with the deepest fundamental Presence of life itself.</u>

> "As your loved one comes closer to his or her death, she may become less
> responsive. Studies indicate that a person ***can still hear*** even if unresponsive,
> so continue to talk to your loved one. Many families find comfort in talking
> about memories that they have about their loved one.
> .....
> ***Gently touch*** your loved one so *your presence* is known... "
>
> [Pathways Hospice, *Guide to Care*, p.17]

Frequently *touch* her hand or her cheek. *Talk* to her. Stay with her. <u>This is the most important time of your marriage</u>.   <u>Your loved one is facing the most profound moment of her life.</u>

<u>She needs her life Partner most at this time</u>

WITH REGARD TO SPIRITUALITY:

Ask if your loved one wants to see a Chaplin, or a Priest, or her Rabbi, or her Imam.   Remind her YOU are here, and will always be with her.   Bring her the sacredness of your life together.

Hospice provides professional palliative end of life care; they are the experts.
They advise Caregivers to

- Maintain a *quiet, peaceful* environment.
- Provide *TOUCH* and reassuring *PRESENCE*;
- *SPEAK* to your loved one---*assume your loved one can hear you.*
  Some things you might want to say are
  "It's okay to let go; I'll (we'll) be all right."
  "I love you."
  If there have been past hurts, then "I forgive you." "Please forgive me."
  [Source: Pathways Hospice, *Dying Is...,* p. 14]

Do not be afraid if she asks tough spiritual questions—"Am I dying?" "Is God really real?"
Answer honestly. <u>Remind her of whatever she has believed all her life</u>....and then urge her to
" <u>let go *fear*,</u>"......"<u>let go *doubt*.</u>"   <u>People tend to die as they have lived</u>.

 Bring her any spiritual remembrance or symbol—like her Bible, or a favorite crucifix, or her mother's locket necklace, or the picture of a child she lost to illness----<u>anything from her life</u> <u>that evokes **a sense of *spirituality* or *beauty*.</u>   Talk to her about what you have brought.

[In our own situation, I brought my dying wife the rosary her mother had left for her when her mother had died of cervical cancer back in 1960. My loved one had cherished it and kept it in a special place. I wrapped it around her hand and invited her to "look for her mother in the Light." I believe it gave her *a place to go*, a *focus* to bridge her transition into death.]

Hospice literature gives anecdotal evidence that the dying frequently see loved ones that have gone ahead, or get a sense of embarking on a long journey.   In the literature of both dying, and out-of-body experiences, a common testimony involves seeing a "Light" and/or meeting loved ones who have gone before.

If your <u>loved one has **not believed in anything beyond death**</u>, do not force anything on her. Tell her she will be "...at Peace," "....at Rest," relieved of all the pain and suffering she is experiencing now.   Remind her of good days, great experiences shared.   Always reassure her that *YOU* are here. *TOUCH* her hand, or her cheek. *TALK* to her; assume she can hear you. Hearing is normally the last physical sense to shut down.

Reassure her "All will be O.K."   Be there for her. Be her Rock.   <u>Give her your Peace.</u>

ABOUT THE AUTHOR

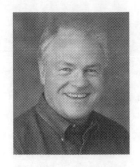

John Garnand has spent a lifetime as a *teacher*.

Most recently, John retired from the Leeds School of Business of the University of Colorado at Boulder.   For twenty-one years, he was an award winning instructor in the general areas of business strategy, management operations, ethics, and public policy.   While at the University, he established the Multicultural Business Students Association, to help disadvantaged students compete and excel.

Before this, Dr. Garnand held the position of Vice President for Administration at Regis University in Denver, CO.   He was also a graduate faculty member in the Regis University Masters of Business Administration (MBA) program.

John Garnand also spent career time in industry, as Corporate Manager of Regulatory Matters at U.S. West Communications. In the capacity of regulatory support he wrote testimony and prepared documentation for State regulatory activities.   He helped implement a competitive markets seminar addressing the issues all managers in the Company would face after the Antitrust breakup of the Bell System.   Dr. Garnand was concurrently a faculty member in the Graduate School of Public Affairs, University of Colorado at Denver.

 Before these assignments, John was a high school teacher, tennis and debate coach.

I believe that lifelong teaching consequently requires lifelong learning. Learning is more than accumulation of facts; it is nurturing the hunger to understand, the yearning for meaning, and resolution of the *whys* of life. In the course of life, there are so many new things to learn every day—if we will be open to their existence and insistence. ***We become what we learn.***

I believe that none of us was fully prepared when the call came to become a Caregiver to our loved one diagnosed with a major disease. **Caregiving is "on-the-job-learning"** and that leads us to the purpose for this book.

This book is my effort to pull together all the information that I have had to learn over nine years of attending to my cancer patient loved one.   It is my hope that this compilation will make it easier for other Cancer Caregivers faced with similar circumstances.

My loved one taught me everything in life that is important to learn. And I now believe that the acquisition of wisdom is just being open to learning, and that anything good that we have learned will never be completely lost. In its existential context *learning defines our lifetime.*

johnjgarnand@gmail.com

JG